Risk and

Sociology and Nursing Practice Series

Davina Allen and David Hughes
Nursing and the Division of Labour in Healthcare

Lorraine Culley and Simon Dyson
Ethnicity and Nursing Practice

Paul Godin
Risk and Nursing Practice

Margaret Miers
Class, Inequalities and Nursing Practice

Margaret Miers
Gender Issues and Nursing Practice

Sam Porter
Social Theory and Nursing Practice

Geoff Wilkinson and Margaret Miers
Power and Nursing Practice

Sociology and Nursing Practice Series
Series Standing Order: ISBN 0–333–69329–9
(*outside North America only*)

You can receive future titles in this series as they are published by placing a standing order. Please contact your bookseller or, in case of difficulty, write to us at the address below with your name and address, the title of the series and the ISBN quoted above.

Customer Services Department, Macmillan Distribution Ltd, Houndmills, Basingstoke, Hampshire RG21 6XS, England

Risk and Nursing Practice

Edited by

Paul Godin

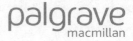

First published 2006 by
PALGRAVE MACMILLAN
Houndmills, Basingstoke, Hampshire RG21 6XS and
175 Fifth Avenue, New York, N.Y. 10010
Companies and representatives throughout the world

PALGRAVE MACMILLAN is the global academic imprint of the Palgrave Macmillan division of St. Martin's Press, LLC and of Palgrave Macmillan Ltd. Macmillan® is a registered trademark in the United States, United Kingdom and other countries. Palgrave is a registered trademark in the European Union and other countries.

ISBN-13: 978–1–4039–4311–8
ISBN-10: 1–4039–4311–7

This book is printed on paper suitable for recycling and made from fully managed and sustained forest sources.

A catalogue record for this book is available from the British Library.

10 9 8 7 6 5 4 3 2 1
15 14 13 12 11 10 09 08 07 06

Printed and bound in China

For Geraldine, Patrick and Tara

Contents

Series editors' preface

It is widely accepted that sociology has the potential to make a significant contribution to nursing's knowledge base. As a discipline it offers valuable and pertinent insights into the causes and distribution of ill health, the experience of health illness and disability, the dynamics of health care encounters and the possibilities and limitations of professional care. In addition, sociology's emphasis on critical reflection encourages nurses to be questioning and self-aware, thus helping them to provide flexible, non-discriminatory, user-centred care in various situations.

Nursing has long been a noteworthy subject for sociological study, both as a developing and changing profession and as an interactive activity between individuals. Sociologists sometimes struggle, however, to offer insights concerning the actual work that nurses do. This is partially due to the limitations of sociological surveillance. Nurses work in confidential, private and intimate settings with their clients. Sociologists' access to such settings is necessarily restricted. Moreover, nurses can find it difficult to talk about their work, except, perhaps to other nurses.

Nursing has a long tradition of drawing on sociology to explore social interaction, particularly to understand social processes such as labeling and stigma. As nursing gains confidence in using and generating research nurse researchers draw increasingly on social science literature to illuminate the restraints and enablements imposed on individual health care interactions by social structures. Nurses are joining multidisciplinary research teams in which nurses and sociologists work together to explore the complexity and dynamics of health and social care policy and practice.

The aim of the *Sociology and Nursing Practice Series* is to support links between the disciplines and to increase nursing and sociology's mutual understanding. The authors of the series' titles and chapters are nurses, teachers of nurses and researchers in health and social care. Together the authors have an intimate understanding of nursing work, an appreciation of the importance of individualised nursing care and a commitment to a sociological outlook that asserts the salience of wider social forces to the work of nurses. The texts apply sociological theories and concepts to practical aspects of nursing. They explore nursing care as part of the social world, showing how different approaches to understanding the relationship between the individual and society have implications for nursing practice. By concentrating on specific concepts and drawing on research informed by social theory and methods, each book is able to provide the reader with a deeper understanding of the social construction of nurses' work.

Risk and Nursing Practice explores ways of understanding risk discourses that identify 'risk' as a central concept in modern society and the management of risk as central to advanced liberalism. As such, discourses about risk have become key to the development and management of health care. The authors demonstrate the relevance of theories about risk to nurses' daily decision making through drawing on their experience of nursing practice and findings from their original research. The chapters clarify how societal processes can restrain nursing practice, but also provide examples of enabling approaches, in which nurses have the confidence to practice therapeutic risk taking. *Risk and Nursing Practice* nurtures a sociological understanding of risk and nursing, more than fulfilling the aims of the book series. We hope reading this book will encourage nurses to analyse critically their practice and profession and to develop their own contribution to health care.

Margaret Miers, Sam Porter, Geoff Wilkinson

Acknowledgements

This book is the result of many people's efforts other than mine. Margaret Miers and Geoff Wilkinson offered advice, support and encouragement throughout. Peggy Drury, Margaret Miers, Jacqueline Davies and two anonymous reviewers read the text assiduously, offering useful comments. The contributing authors, Andy Alaszewski, Mary Ann Elston, Jonathan Gabe, Maria O'Beirne, Karen Mackinnon, Liza McCoy, David Pontin, Bob Heyman, Jacqueline Davies and Anthony Pryce, have provided excellent chapters exploring risk and nursing practice in a broad range of situations. Lynda Thompson and her colleagues at Palgrave have provided a high standard of editorial guidance and support.

Finally I would like to thank my wife Geraldine for her help, support and understanding of her husband too often in front of the computer.

Paul Godin

Paul Godin, Jacqueline Davies and Bob Heyman would like to thank the patients and staff of unit featured within their study for their participation within the research.

Andy Alaszewski would like to thank the English National Board for Nursing, Midwifery and health visiting for permission to reprint material from Table 2.1 and Table 3.1 from Andy Alaszewski *et al. Assessing and Managing Risk in Nursing Education and Practice: Supporting Vulnerable People in the Community*, 1998.

Karen MacKinnon would like to thank her friends and colleagues Merry Little, Margaret Quance, Julianne Sanguins and Donna Wallace for their thoughtful review and feedback on an earlier draft of 'The very LOUD Discourses of Risk in Pregnancy'.

Notes on contributors

Andy Alaszewski is Professor of Health Studies and Director of the Centre for Health Services Research at the University of Kent. In the last ten years he has examined the ways in which the assessment, perception and management of risk structures the ways in which service users experience the care and support they receive. He has recently completed a methodological text for Sage on *Using Diaries for Social Research* (2005) and is editor of *Health, Risk and Society*.

Jacqueline Davies is Research Fellow in the Health Care Research Unit at the St Bartholomew School of Nursing and Midwifery, City University, London. Since undertaking the research discussed in Chapter 5 and Chapter 8 of this book, she has worked with Godin, Heyman and others developing further research projects in the area of forensic mental health investigating: service-user-led research, the experiences of family carers and inpatient care in South Africa.

Mary Ann Elston was Reader in Medical Sociology at Royal Holloway, and is currently Visiting Reader in Sociology at the University of Surrey. Her research interests are in the sociology of health care work and organisations, particularly in gender and the health professions. She has recently edited *Key Concepts and Issues in the Sociology of Health and Illness* (2004) for Sage with Jonathan Gabe and Mike Bury.

Jonathan Gabe is Reader in Sociology in the Department of Health and Social Care, Royal Holloway, University of London. He is co-editor (with Stefan Timmermans) of *Partners in Health, Partners in Crime. Exploring the Boundaries of Criminology and Sociology of Health and Illness* (2003), published by Blackwell. He has particular interests in violence against health care professionals, and in health care organisation and chronic illness.

Paul Godin is Senior Lecturer in Sociology at St Bartholomew School of Nursing and Midwifery, City University, London. His research activities have involved investigating the work of community mental health care nurses and forensic mental health care, which he has used to inform Chapter 4 and Chapter 5. In a year-long Department of Health funded project, from 2004 to 2005, Paul was the principal investigator of a team that enabled forensic mental health care service users to undertake research evaluation of their care. He has published a number of papers in nursing and inter-professional journals, and contributed chapters to books, such as *Class and Nursing Practice*, edited by Margaret Miers (2003), published by Palgrave.

Bob Heyman is Associate Dean for Research and Professor of Health Research at St Bartholomew School of Nursing and Midwifery, City University. He has a longstanding interest in qualitative approaches to health risk management, and has been undertaking research on this issue in various clinical settings, including forensic mental health care, support for adults with learning disabilities and prenatal chromosomal screening, for many years. He has authored two books in this field, *Risk, Health and Health Care: A Qualitative Approach* (1997) for Hodder Arnold, and *Risk, Age and Pregnancy* (2001) for Palgrave.

Khim Horton is Post Doctoral Research Fellow at the Centre for Research in Nursing and Midwifery Education, European Institute of Health and Medical Sciences, University of Surrey. She is a qualified nurse with expertise in the care of older people. She is also actively involved with the British Society of Gerontology.

Liza McCoy is Assistant Professor of Sociology at the University of Calgary. Her research interests are in the areas of health and employment. She has recently studied the health work of people living with HIV and is currently researching the experience of immigrant women seeking to re-establish careers in non-regulated professional occupations.

Karen MacKinnon, a certified Perinatal Nurse, recently completed her PhD examining the social determinants of women's preterm labour experiences at the University of Calgary. Karen is currently building a research programme that focuses on social justice issues affecting women's childbearing experiences and perinatal nursing practice. She has also been involved in research about women's experiences of the nurse's presence during childbirth; the effects of hydrotherapy (water immersion) on women's discomfort/labour pain; continuity of care; early postpartum discharge and infant crying.

Maria O'Beirne is Honary Research Associate in the Department of Social and Political Science, Royal Holloway, University of London. She has published papers on researching violence in health care and probation settings and is currently completing a doctoral thesis on the role of receptionists in general practice.

David Pontin is Director of Post-graduate Research Studies/Principal Lecturer in Children's Nursing at the University of the West of England (UWE), Bristol. His research activity has focused on the use of action research and qualitative methods of inquiry to address professional practice issues. David is currently working on Community Children's Nursing Caseload issues, nursing care delivery to children and child health issues. He is very closely involved in the MSc Advanced Practice programme at UWE, as well as teaching on child health issues in undergraduate programmes and supervising research degree students. In addition to research papers, David has published research methodology chapters in textbooks such as Cormack [2000] *The Research Process in Nursing*, published by Blackwell Science.

Anthony Pryce is Reader in Sociology of sexual health at City University, London and Honorary Research Fellow at University of Kent. He is currently developing a research programme that addresses a range of projects around marginalised groups, sexualities and sexual health including migrants, sex workers, older people as well as the emergence of the Internet as an arena for developing sexual identities and practices. Anthony is also involved with international projects in Laos and Australia. He has contributed to a number of books; most recently to *Representing Health: Discourses of health and* *illness in the media*, edited by Martin King and Katherine Watson (2005), published by Palgrave.

Professor Monica Shaw was previously Dean of Social Sciences at Northumbria University and is currently part-time Senior Research Fellow at City University. She has written in the past on nursing relationships at work with Heyman and is currently focussing on the challenges of multidisciplinary teamwork in forensic mental health.

1 Introduction

Paul Godin

The word 'risk' now pervades discourses of health and nursing. 'Risk assessment' and 'risk management' have become insistent imperatives, which shape a diverse range of health care and nursing practice. Dowie (1999) contends that this widespread discourse of risk restricts rather than improves our thinking about all that surrounds the term (accident prevention, health promotion, safe clinical practice and so on). 'Risk', he argues, is a conceptual pollutant that encourages us to assume that we know what we are talking about when we do not. We use the term simultaneously as a synonym for both probability and harm, and make little distinction between actions and out-comes, such that the effective utility of the term is seriously limited. Dowie suggests that our decision making in matters of health, would improve were we to be more circumspect about our acceptance and use of the word 'risk'. However, the varied and widespread use of the word risk begs the question, 'how has such diverse and widespread use of the term arisen?' And, what have been its social consequences, other than to simply confuse our thinking? These are sociological questions that this book goes some way towards answering.

In this book sociological insights are employed to understand risk in its various forms of discourse and associated practices, within some of the many arenas in which nursing takes place. At a general level, risk management has become an integral part of nursing. The Nursing and Midwifery Council (NMC) advise that 'The risk management process should enable the optimum level of care to be given to a client' (NMC 2004a). Nurses can thereby discharge their responsibility, under clause 1.3 of the 'NMC Code of professional conduct', to be personally accountable for their practice.

Though nurses and other health care professionals have long been concerned with their responsibility towards patients in the face of clinical uncertainty about various forms of care and treatment, there is now a heightened emphasis upon individual accountability, given by the discourse of risk. In a questionnaire and interview study of legal accountability, Annandale (1996) found that nurses spoke of experiencing risk as something that, for them, looms large and continuously in the background. In a climate of risk they feared being identified as having made a mistake, which would result in blame and litigation (described by one nurse as a 'bogey man'). Nurses commonly stated that they thought this climate of risk had arisen as a consequence of patients becoming more aware of their rights than ever before and therefore more likely to pursue litigation. A feeling of vulnerability stood like an omnipresent cloud hanging over nurses' daily practice. They spoke of how they anxiously sought to manage and avert future potential problems and crises through such measures as keeping accurate and detailed records. A ward sister described how a junior colleague 'was coming in on days off on a *pretence* that she was visiting, just to make sure that she'd done everything and that she wasn't in trouble' (1996: 429). For many nurses, their anxiety and sense of vulnerability was compounded by experiences of having little control and being unsupported by their management. Above all, Annandale's study demonstrates how although nursing discourse emphasises the facilitative role of the nurse, engaged in a partnership of care with the patient; the patient as a consumer is perceived as someone who generates risk. Rather than feeling intimately engaged in close trusting therapeutic relationships with patients, nurses spoke of often feeling like airhostesses, insincerely smiling at their customers, whilst sometimes wanting to scream at them. In Chapter 3, Elston *et al.*, revisit Annandale's idea of the patient as a risk generating demanding consumer, explaining that as such they might well become angry or aggressive towards National Health Service (NHS) staff. Elston *et al.*, point to how a number of writers have identified this as the reason why nurses and health care policy makers have become increasingly concerned about patients being violent towards NHS staff.

The intrusion of risk management into nursing and health care more generally is also apparent in an increasing number of textbooks for health care professionals on the subject. In *Risk Management in Healthcare* Roberts and Holly attempt to convince their readers of the vital importance and need for risk management in health care, asserting that 'A good understanding of how to deal with risk can mean the difference between the success and the failure of the single clinical episode and of the healthcare services as a whole' (1996: 1).

The discourse of risk management features ever more prominently in health care policy, instructing NHS employees to undertake risk assessment and risk management in their practice. New Labour NHS policy has inaugurated a 'National Patient Safety Agency' to attend to the risks that patients face in receiving care. In *Building a safer NHS for patients* (Department of Health (DoH) 2000a) it is asserted that the NHS could usefully emulate the practices of the aviation industry that attempt to amass information about crashes and near misses to analyse and learn from such mistakes. Specific risks have been targeted for action, such as the reduction in drug errors and the elimination of suicides amongst mental health in-patients. New posts have been created within the NHS, such as 'clinical risk managers' to lead this project in the rational control of risk, towards the improvement of health care. The NMC list risk management, alongside evidence-based practices, as a 'quality improvement initiative' that should, they advise, be co-ordinated within clinical governance (NMC 2004b). However, though risk management discourse is primarily about avoiding injury and loss in health care delivery, it is only the tip of the iceberg of risk discourse within health care.

Risk discourse features prominently in the discourse of health promotion, which has become an ever more significant part of health care practices. The project of health promotion, articulated in *The Health of the Nation* (DoH 1992), *Saving Lives: Our Healthier Nation* (DoH 1999a) and *Chosing Health: making healthier choices easier* (DoH 2004a) now drives NHS policy. A primary objective of this calculative and rational project is to reduce the risk/incidence of diseases through preventive measures. It is indicative of a shift in health care that Armstrong (1995) argues involves a re-mapping of illness. 'Hospital Medicine', he contends, involves identifying, categorising and curing illness within individual patients. 'Surveillance Medicine', that is now surpassing Hospital Medicine, involves the dissolution of the distinct clinical categories of health and illness to bring the entire population into the clinical gaze. Under this new regime, medicine concentrates upon identifying and attending to 'risk factors', from which a probability of illness can be calculated. As Armstrong explains 'illness is simply a nodal point in a network of health status monitoring' (1995: 401). The massive workforce of NHS nurses plays a substantial part in sustaining this network of risk factor monitoring, from health visitors carrying out developmental tests on children, to practice nurses undertaking routine health checks on older adults.

Apart from inspiring nurses to save themselves and the NHS from litigation, and their patients from iatrogenic treatment and potential ill health in the future, health policy risk discourse also demands a safe working environment within the NHS, which has been declared a 'zero tolerance zone' (ZTZ) with respect to violence from the public (NHS Executive 2001a). Though, as we have seen from Annandale's study, nurses may fear patient consumers as generators of risk, the government has, seemingly, introduced this measure to ensure that the demands of patient consumers do not erupt into violence against staff. Chapter 3 deals with the risk of violence against nurses and health service staff in some depth.

So far I have considered only how the discourse of risk generated by health policy has shaped nursing practices. However, this is not the only source from which risk discourse in health care flows. Skolbekken (1995) traces the rise in 'risk articles' (articles with risk in their title) within medical journals published from 1967 to 1991 in the United States of America, Britain and Scandinavia. He identifies an accelerating increase in risk articles, particularly within epidemiological journals, outstripping the general rise in the number of published articles, which he likens to an 'epidemic'. Speculating as to the cause of this epidemic, he suggests that the development of computer technology, allowing advanced statistical analysis calculations, to assist quantitative research studies may have been a contributing factor. He also speculates that the rise of health promotion and a growing concern of medicine to identify risk factors of disease (what Armstrong terms Surveillance Medicine) might also have played a part. Skolbekken then pertinently notes that the risk epidemic does not reflect an enlarged danger to our health, as there has been a marked increase in life expectancy in the Western world. Finally, he cautions against possible harmful effects of the risk epidemic, namely defensive medical practice that prevents positive risk taking and the imposition of an unhealthy preoccupation with potential diseases amongst healthy people.

Using the 'Cumulative Index to Nursing & Allied Health Literature' (CINAHL) database, I emulated Skolbekken's exercise to see whether a risk epidemic had also affected nursing journals. Skolbekken notes a rise in the percentage of risk articles within generalist medical journals from 0.1 per cent in the 1967–1971 period to between 4 per cent and 10 per cent in the 1982–1986 period, and to between 6.5 per cent and 12 per cent in the 1987–1991 period. As CINAHL only listed articles from 1982 my historical search was limited to this point. In the 1982–1986 period, there was a less than 1 per cent rate of risk articles in the following generalist nursing journals: *Journal of Advanced Nursing, International Journal of Nursing Studies* and the *Nursing Times*. The rate remained at this low level for subsequent years in most of these journals, only getting to rates of 2 per cent or 3 per cent in the Journal of Advanced Nursing and the International Journal of Nursing during the twenty-first century; hardly enough to be described as an epidemic. However, as Elston *et al.*, demonstrate in Chapter 3, there has been a substantial growth in the last 20 years of risk articles about violence of patients and the public towards nurses.

Though risk discourse might be less prevalent within nursing journals than medical journals, as the subsequent chapters of this book demonstrate, risk discourse is otherwise widely apparent within nursing. Why should this be? I suggest that this recent preoccupation with risk is not confined to nursing or health care alone, but is more widely apparent within contemporary society. Therefore, to develop a sociological understanding of risk and nursing practice requires a consideration of how social theorists have endeavoured to understand how and why society has become preoccupied with risk. To this end I now outline three major approaches of social theory that variously attempt to understand this phenomenon. First, I consider how sociologists, such as Beck and Giddens, explain how structures and processes of late modernity give rise to what Beck calls 'risk society'. Second, I consider how anthropologists, such as Douglas, explain how culture shapes our cognition and selection of risk, and our behaviour towards it. Last, I consider how Foucault's theory of governmentality has been applied to understand how discourses and practices around risk give rise to a particular form of subjectivity and liberal rule. These perspectives reappear in the following chapters, along with other social theory, towards developing a sociological understanding of risk and nursing practice.

The 'risk society' approach

Beck (1992) coined the term 'risk society' as a descriptor of contemporary western society, which he believed to be in a transitional period within modernity. He argues that in pre-modern society, plague, famine, natural catastrophes and the other such threats it faced were deemed incalculable and attributed to supernatural causes. Through industrialisation, early modernity took shape in the nineteenth century and transformed the threats of pre-modern society, through rational control, into calculable risks. Beck contends that we have now moved into a transitional era in which the processes of modernist risk calculation fail. In 'risk society' the hazards we face are largely the product of modernity, as scientific and industrial development increasingly threaten the environment. These risks are often invisible, unknowable and not easily calculable. For example, the future effect of global warming cannot be determined. Furthermore, the effects of these new hazards, as Chernobyl illustrates, can be global, long-lasting and irreparable. Scientific industrialised modernity that once controlled risk, has produced a new range of hazards, of a potentially cataclysmic nature. The claims of experts to knowledge about these new hazards contradict each other and experts cannot be relied upon to provide solutions to the problems these hazards create. Whereas knowledge reduced uncertainty in early modernity, uncertainty has now arisen out of the growth of knowledge in late modernity. Giddens (1991: 3) makes a similar point in his description of the 'risk culture' of late modernity. He explains that exposure to danger, and anxiety about it, is not peculiar to our time. However, that danger is now seen as having been brought about by humans, rather than the gods or fate, is unique to late modernity, what Giddens calls its 'dark side'.

Beck argues that the modern age was characterised by a class structure that took form out of industrial capitalism, giving rise to the production and inequitable distribution of goods. In late modernity, capitalism has taken a new form, eroding production-based class identity. The central problem of late modernity is less about the production and distribution of goods but more about the prevention or minimisation of bads. The hazards late modernity produces are distributed somewhat differently than is wealth within modern society, as they can potentially affect rich and poor alike. Thus Beck writes 'poverty is hierarchic, smog is democratic' (1992: 36), though he does clearly acknowledge that the poor generally endure a greater amount of bads. However, Beck emphasises that this inequality is not a mere correlate of class, for class society has given way to risk society.

Beck elaborates two further inter-related concepts that are central to his view of the risk society. First, he argues that a surge of 'individualization' has occurred within late modernity. It has been brought about by the fragmenting effect of globalisation, eroding national and cultural boundaries, and a reduced influence of traditional structuring institutions, such as the family, the welfare state, traditional industries and class-based political parties. This disintegration of the traditional leads to uncertainty amongst people who find themselves free from traditional constraints and free to shape their own destiny. We have thus become individualised by late modernity, anxiously seeking and inventing new certainties. We are forced to construct our own biographies without the guidance of the norms and expectations that emanated from modernity's traditional institutions. Yet in late modernity we are expected to be self-reliant. We, alone, are now seen as largely responsible for our fate and the misfortunes that beset us, for we are expected to seek knowledge about risks and to manage them rationally in our lives. Poverty and unemployment are seen as individual personal problems rather than socially based. Beck's analysis is largely at an abstract and macro-level, and perhaps produces a too over-generalised, rationalistic and individualistic model of human actors. Lash (2000) points out that people do not always rationally seek to avert risk, as they often take risks for pleasure, excitement and self-fulfilment. Tulloch and Lupton (2003) have made an interesting attempt to test out Beck's thesis. In-depth interviews with a cross section of 60 people in Britain and 74 people in Australia were used to explore people's understandings of the concept of risk and how they saw it affecting their lives and those of their compatriots. Though people were found to express anxiety and uncertainty about the future, they were generally less concerned about risks that technology inflicts upon the environment than they were about crime and a dystopic future of social disorder. However, those with greater wealth and power expressed greater personal optimism about their ability to cope within a changing world. Those in less-advantaged positions more readily saw the risks and uncertainties they faced as being socially produced and requiring of government interventions. Tulloch and Lupton found that their interviewees' reflexive responses to risk were strongly shaped by gender, age, occupation, nationality and sexual identity. Though Beck might be correct in suggesting that the surge of individualisation has occurred, he is, perhaps, wrong to suggest that people respond to it in a uniform manner. Seemingly, structure and/or culture shape a variety of understandings and responses to risk. As I later explain, the anthropologist Mary Douglas provides key insights about how culture can be understood variously to affect people's risk thinking and behaviour.

Second, Beck argues rather optimistically, that risk society is accompanied by 'reflexive modernization'. The risks of late modern society serve to pose questions about current practices as modernity comes to examine and critique itself.

Just as Enlightenment demystified and overturned a religious worldview and pre-modern order, so too is reflexive modernity questioning the principles and organisation of industrial society, towards the creation of a new order. Beck explains 'we are witnessing not the end but the *beginning* of modernity – that is, of a modernity *beyond* its classical industrial design' (1992: 10). Other writers such as Giddens (1991) and Lash (1992) have more fully developed the concept of reflexivity in late modern society. Giddens emphasises that it is a monitoring process of self and others, made possible by an implosion of information systems. As information about our world becomes more available, we become saturated with it. It can bear down heavily on us as a source of constant worry. Applying this concept to the findings of her own study, Annanandale (1996) speculates that the patient as consumer, exposed to news reports about NHS financial cutbacks, bungled operations and incompetent practice, are therefore anxious about their care and feel a need to question and challenge health care professionals. The professional responsibility of nurses and other health care professionals towards their patients is, perhaps, intensified by what Beck identifies as 'individualization' and by what Giddens describes as the condition of the risk culture of reflexive modernity, in which the future has to be continually drawn into the present to avert risk. Thus professionals feel compelled to do all they anxiously can to manage risks in order to avert hazards and so avoid the accompanying bogey man of blame and litigation.

This risk society/risk culture theoretical approach, that I have just outlined, has had a considerable influence on New Labour policy. On the back cover of *The Third Way* (Giddens 1998) it is noted that Giddens has been described as Tony Blair's 'guru' and 'favourite intellectual'. The book is an attempt to make theoretical sense of and justify third way politics. It does so by explaining how globalisation and risk society/risk culture require the state to take a new role, enabling citizens to successfully adapt, as active individuals, to the changing world of reflexive modernity, in which traditional institutions have been lost. Giddens recommends that the state should encourage a new type of civilised individualism, distinctly different from the selfish individualism of the

Thatcher/Major era. He talks of a need to 'reconstruct' the welfare state, rather than rebuilding it in its traditional form, through 'positive welfare'. As Giddens explains

> Positive welfare would replace each of Beveridge's negatives with a positive: in place of Want, autonomy; not Disease but active health; instead of Ignorance, education, as a continuing part of life; rather than Squalor, well-being; and in place of Idleness, initiative. (1998: 128)

Therefore, in this age of reflexive modernity, New Labour policy attempts to encourage us all to actively improve our own welfare and human capacity, with the assistance of an enabling, rather than providing, state, to avert the risk of individual and social failure. As Higgs (1998) points out citizenship is thus being reconceptualised. It is no longer based on our membership of a collectivity but is now becoming a set of procedural rights and duties with which individuals are exhorted to comply. Without elaborating detail of all such New Labour policy it is perhaps sufficient to say that policy in the areas of health and education have had most influence on nurses. New Labour policy has advanced projects of patient safety and health promotion, encouraging vigilant risk management amongst health professionals and the active pursuit of good health among all good citizens. Education and 'life long learning' have been declared essential for an adaptive and effective workforce. The government boasts about the increasing number of doctors and nurses it is training and how post-qualification education of health professionals is encouraged through such initiatives as the NHS Institute for Learning, Skills and Innovation (formerly the NHS University). Thus, the risk society approach is more than just a theory. As an ideology it has influenced government thinking and policy to have an effect upon the working lives of nurses.

The cultural approach

The anthropologist Mary Douglas has been the main exponent of the sociocultural analysis of risk. Her interest in risk grew out of her earlier work that considered how contamination and danger were socially regulated (Douglas 1966). She makes continual comparisons between how danger is understood within primitive cultures and how risk is understood within modern society, highlighting both similarities and differences. The term 'risk', Douglas (1990) argues, arose in the seventeenth century when it was associated with gambling and games of chance, the study of which led to a special branch of mathematics, statistics. In modern society, interest in risk has become more generalised, becoming central to our thinking and behaviour. Douglas (1992) contends that the term risk within a global society, because of its scientificity and connection with objective analysis, provides an inter-community discourse. As 'modern' people we commonly think that our concept of risk makes us distinctly different from 'primitive' and 'pre-modern' people, who explain misfortunes as the result of the sins of those who are beset by them. However, Douglas points out that in a similar fashion risk allows blame to be attributed, for she says of risk 'Above all, its forensic uses fit the tool to the task of building a culture that supports a modern industrial society' (1992: 15). In contemporary western culture almost every accident, death, sickness or other misfortune becomes chargeable to someone's account in a new blaming system. Blame is as culturally functional to modern culture, with its risk discourse, as the identification of sin is within primitive and pre-modern cultures. Being 'at risk' is the modern equivalent of being sinned against. The practice of establishing who is good or bad and who is at fault is key to maintaining the organisation of all cultures. For all its scientific and value free appearance, risk is a forensic device, used moralistically and politically. Whereas Beck shows how the conditions of late modernity produce a particular type of hazard/risk and an individualised and reflexive response to it, Douglas endeavours to understand risk as a socially constructed interpretation and reaction to dangers that is suitable for modern society.

Douglas particularly draws our attention to the ways in which our thinking about risk, and cognition more generally, is socially constructed within the institutions and cultures of which we are part. She is repeatedly critical of psychologists and economists who portray cognition and risk perception as private, individual and rational. That people perceive risk differently is based less on their intellectual ability to think rationally than on the prejudices of the institutions to which they are committed. As Douglas put it:

> individuals do not try to make independent choices, especially about big political issues. When faced with estimating probability and credibility, they come already primed with culturally learned assumptions and weightings. (1992: 58)

In *Risk and Culture*, Douglas and Wildavsky (1983) consider whether there could be any way of assessing and ranking the dangers we face, in order of their threat to us, to carry out the objective risk assessment and management of risk. Such a project, they argue, is doomed for two reasons.

First, nobody can know more than a fraction of the dangers that abound. Our position cannot be improved by gaining more scientific knowledge, for the more we learn the more we become aware of what we don't know and cannot be sure of, and the more uncertain we become about what is and is not a danger to us.

Second, we could not avoid representing particular interests about what matters, what is desirable and who should rule. In other words, the project could not avoid being political. Thus we culturally select the risks we choose to attend to and those that we choose to ignore. The choices we make in our selection may appear irrational to those who do not share our prejudices and values. The outsider might observe that we seek to protect 'unimportant' things whilst ignoring that which threatens our very existence. Douglas and Wildavsky (1983) illustrate this through presenting hypothetical dialogues that might occur between a western scientist and a Hima nomad. Each, as an outsider to the other's culture, would see the other's prioritisation of risk as irrational. Yet that which threatens our culture is not unimportant. Culture is our way of maintaining an ordered understanding of our world, such that we can operate within it. Therefore, threats to culture are often prioritised as risks of paramount importance, above threats to our physical existence, precisely because in a different way, they also threaten our existence. To illustrate the point within a contemporary context, consider the issue of global warming. Greens shout loudly that continuation of current methods of production and use of energy have already created millions of 'environmental refugees', from desertification, rising sea levels and shrinking freshwater supplies; a trend that threatens to soon render our planet entirely uninhabitable. Does this persuade us, in the industrialised world, to stop flying in aeroplanes, driving cars and doing all the other things that are integral to our lives and may also ultimately result in the demise of humankind? We cannot make the changes that are necessary to avert disaster without radically changing our cultural way of life, a task that is, perhaps, beyond us. Therefore, we continue to destroy the conditions that are necessary for our existence. We avoid the risk of having to change our way of lives, ignoring the disastrous not too long-term risk; a risk that we can never have full knowledge of and can, therefore, choose to perceive as uncertain and unreal.

Douglas and Wildavsky (1983) also point out that it is mistaken to assume that the elimination of risk only gets rid of that which is undesirable, for as they explain: 'Life's choices, after all, often come as a bundle of goods and bads, which have to be taken whole' (1983: 18). For example, the goods of industrial society comes with bads, such as the potential loss of human habitation on Earth. Risks are often accompanied with rewards that may be forgone if risks are not taken. Thus, as a number of the chapters within this book illustrate, risk management strategies that ensure patients' safety are often achieved at the expense of patients' autonomy and enjoyment of life.

The influence of Durkheim is extremely evident in Douglas's work. As Durkheim attempted to understand suicide in terms of how people are integrated and regulated into society, Douglas attempts to understand how people's risk perceptions and related behaviour are also influenced by their integration and regulation into society. In a shorthand fashion, she refers to integration as 'group' and regulation as 'grid'. Douglas and Wildavsky provide clarity of meaning to these terms as follows:

> *Group* means the outside boundary that people have erected between themselves and the outside world. *Grid* means all the other social distinctions and delegations of authority that they use to limit how people behave to one another. (1983: 138)

Based on these two dimensions Douglas constructs a grid/group model to understand how people, organisations and cultures develop different understandings and approaches to risk. Though she applies this grid/group model in the analysis of a wide range of situations the most relevant illustration for the purpose of this book is, perhaps, that of the City (a term used to refer broadly to the culture of western society) dealing with the threat of AIDS, when the pandemic first arose in the mid-1980s. Douglas describes four ideal type positions of grid and group.

First, in the high grid/high group position, the hierarchically structured city core or central community attempted to defend itself against those it identifies as deviant outsiders (gays and drug users) who transgressed its norms and values. To control this risk, the central community re-asserted its moral order, reinforcing its boundaries to exclude outsiders, who were seen as contagious others. This identification of otherness helped build social solidarity within the central community.

Second, in the low grid/high group position, a dissenting enclave of homosexuals, united by the central community's marginalisation of them, rejected the moral and social order that portrayed them as the 'at risk' group of denizens. They challenged their 'at risk' status and the central community's knowledge base and authority, advancing alternative ideas as to the cause of AIDS and how it could be effectively treated.

Third, in the low grid/low group position individuals ('cultural frontiersmen', entrepreneurs, and professionals) took risks for the advantages that they may afford, trusting to luck. The character Roy Cohn, played by Al Pacino, in the television drama '*Angels in America*' epitomises the cultural frontiersmen/entrepreneur. Medical professionals took risks, as autonomous leaders of the central community, supplying it with authoritative knowledge about AIDS.

Last, in the high grid/low group position, isolates (drug addicts, prostitutes and loners), expelled from the central community, constitute a residual category of people whose autonomy has been withdrawn from them. Powerless to resist their at risk status, they were also exposed to risks, which they endured with a fatalistic attitude.

Chapter Five revisits this grid/group model, drawing parallels between the City dealing with AIDS and the present day City dealing with the deinstitutionalised madness to consider how staff within a forensic mental health care variously recognise and deal with the risk they are charged with controlling.

The governmentality approach

Having described modern society as 'disciplinary' and 'carceral', in his later work, Foucault advances the concept of 'governmentality' to identify another form of power that operates within the modern era. Foucault (1991) draws attention to how, in Sixteenth- and Seventeenth-century Europe, writings about the 'art of government' became less concerned with the conduct and behaviour of the sovereign, and more concerned with the 'right disposition of things', the economy and the population. Government became less concerned with the imposition of law and more concerned with the implementation of strategy and rationale. The rise of political economy and 'police' (not in the sense of 'police force' but in the sense of 'policy') were symptomatic of this change. The population was increasingly understood as something requiring measurement, management and protection in order to maximise its productivity, wealth, health and welfare. As Foucault explains 'population comes to appear above all else as the ultimate end of government' (1991: 100). In developing strategies and policies to attend to the population, the state became 'governmentalized'.

A number of writers have attempted to develop Foucault's concept of governmentality, to understand how this population focused form of power has taken shape in more recent times and how, in particular, the concept of risk has become a central feature within it. Though there are differences between these writers, they all regard government as something that is not limited to the confines of the state apparatus. Thereby, they distance themselves from the previous generation of Marxists writers who understood the state to be an instrumental means of power to support class domination within capitalism. Marxists commonly regard the rise of risk discourse within health care as one of many forms of capitalist ideology that function to individualise the causes of ill health, poverty and other misfortunes which, they argue, are in fact brought about by capitalism. White, for example, argues

> When epidemiologists focus on the proximate causes of disease, diet, cholesterol and hypertension, for example, they individualize the causes of disease and miss the distal social causes ... we need to con-textualize risk factors so as to see how individuals are exposed to them and have limited access to resources to respond to them. (2002: 62)

However, Marxists frequently provide somewhat abstract and functionalist accounts of how capitalism causes disease and creates its particular organisational system of health care. Rather than looking to the context of the economic class system to understand the causes of disease and why health care operates as it does, the new generation of governmentality theorists look to understand how society's pervasive political rationality of liberalism, with its powerful risk discourse, gives rise to a collection of programmes, technologies and practices through which health care policy and practice is governed.

Castel (1991), Rose (1993) and Dean (1997) all draw attention to the way in which rationalities and technologies of risk figure prominently in western society's contemporary style of liberal rule, which they refer to as either 'advanced liberalism' or 'neo-liberalism'. Whereas the risk society approach asserts that it is the conditions of late modernity with its frightening mega hazards, that give rise to our present obsession with risk, governmentality theorists argue rather that it is through the discourses and practices of contemporary liberal rule that we come to be preoccupied with risk, as something to be problematised, rendered calculable and governable.

Governmentality theorists attempt to understand how advanced liberalism operates through tracing the historical development of liberalism. Rose (1993) argues that liberalism inaugurated a continuing questioning of the activity of rule, which promoted the transformation from one problematic of rule to the next. Rose explains that liberalism is a 'mentality of rule', a political rationality, a way of problematising life which gives rise to particular technologies and practices of rule that bring about governmentality. Though liberalism supports a continuing extension of the rule of the population, it simultaneously limits the scope of political authority to do so by the values it promotes concerning market freedom, civil society and citizenship. Therefore, because of this profoundly moral character liberal governmentality does not involve the total administration of the society.

Different eras of liberalism may be identified by changes in both the mentality and practices of rule. Nineteenth- and early twentieth-century liberalism stressed the values of individualism, laissez-faire economics and social Darwinism, in which welfare was minimal and of a charitable nature. However, this approach became discredited in the face of social fragmentation and the economic depression of the 1930s. The welfare state arose as a formula for the better management of social and economic affairs. In turn, welfare liberalism lost its appeal. Dean (1997) argues that this can be identified within a number of emerging critiques that, during the 1960s and 1970s, drew attention to the controlling, paternalist and patriarchal nature of the state and its professionals. Advanced liberalism (or neo-liberalism) promotes a renewed emphasis on the self, self-reliance and a concern to manage risk.

Rule under any of these forms of liberalism, least of all advanced liberalism, is not reducible to any single clearly definite political ideology and associated practices. As Dean says of advanced liberalism: 'It operates rather through a multiplicity of "practices of freedom," of ways of structuring, shaping, predicting and making calculable, the operation of choice' (1997: 216). Advanced liberalism evokes a considerable amount of subjective self-government. Individuals are encouraged to be autonomous, self-regulating, rational, prudent, entrepreneurial and relentlessly in search of self-improvement. The discourse of risk features prominently in this self-government. We are exhorted to be aware of information about risks to our health and to utilise this knowledge to regulate our diet and lifestyle. Fat people, heavy smokers and those that drink alcohol excessively, are deemed irrational or incapable of self-regulation. Therefore, the project of maintaining one's health is a moral enterprise in which the individual must be eternally vigilant in the avoidance of risk to his/her health. In short, advanced liberalism's emphasis on individual freedom imparts a considerable amount of responsibility on people to rationally manage their own health, welfare, education and general well-being. Integral to such self-management is the expectation of the individual to calculate and manage risk.

Advanced liberalism has also rendered the expert governable. Their autonomy that once distinguished them as professionals has been considerably eroded. For as Castel (1991) argues, in the case of mental health care, professional knowledge increasingly informs the operation of the administrative system above professionals such that control passes to this higher level and professionals become its functionaries. However, it is not that health care professionals have become deprofessionalised within a health care system that has become ever more like Weber's ideal typical bureaucracy. Rather, as Osborne (1993) and Flynn (2002) point out, health care professionals have been co-opted into managerial and clinical rationalities of audit, self-assessment, performance appraisal, risk management and clinical governance; none of which have fully routinised the work of professionals. Thus, in health care, both individual patients and professionals play a full and active part in the creation and operation of the government of themselves.

Health care has developed distinctively risk focused methods of practice within advanced liberalism. As Armstrong (1995) proposes that Hospital Medicine is being surpassed by risk focused Surveillance Medicine, Castel (1991) similarly argues that 'clinic of the subject' is transforming into the risk-oriented 'epidemiological clinic'. Tracing the history of psychiatry in western society, Castel posits that the threat of madness, once thought of as dangerousness, dwelling within the individual mental patients, is now understood as an objective entity, namely risk, existing within the population. Whereas the former understanding gave rise to the asylum system, which simply confined the threat of madness, the latter results in a more proactive monitoring and control of risk to prevent the eruption of madness.

Castel's thesis is widely applicable to all areas of health care within advanced liberalism, as he asserts that a proliferation of health checks has resulted in face-to-face clinical encounters becoming less significant than the health care system's concern to monitor health within the entire population. Health promotion targets to reduce rates of particular diseases are a clear example of this trend towards an epidemiological clinic in which the population, rather than the subject, is regarded as the end of health care strategies. Castel proposes that in such a regime the subject is 'dissolved' as examination of the physically present subject is replaced by examination of records and the control of risk within the population. Health care is practised increasingly at a distance, through such schemes as 'NHS Direct' that reduces face-to-face contact between the subject and the clinician. Lupton (1995) points out that whereas epidemiology was once applied in public health strategies to change the environment, now epidemiological risk factors are used to exhort individuals to regulate their health. Mass-targeted media campaigns encourage individuals to identify themselves as being 'at risk' of heart disease or some other condition and accordingly to take steps to voluntarily reduce their risk.

Nevertheless, the rise of the epidemiological clinic does not mean that face-to-face contact between health care workers and individual subjects has almost disappeared. As Dean points out (1997), sub-populations, such as the 'seriously mentally ill', become identified as 'at risk' and in need of intensive face-to-face case-management. At risk people typically have a limited capacity to manage their lives, in the way advanced liberalism encourages, and are usually socially marginalised. They receive intensive case management, such as 'assertive community treatment' to neutralise or lower the risk they pose to themselves and others. This might involve various forms of therapy, training and detention. The risk discourse that pervades health or social care now overshadows the concept of need. People are perceived as requiring care as a result of their risk status rather than the needs they have. The former is simply assumed to incorporate the latter.

Clearly, governmentality theorists consider similar phenomena to that which Beck and Giddens describe as individualisation and reflexive modernity. However, as I have explained, there are major theoretical differences between these two approaches. Yet, like the risk society approach theorists, governmentality theorists have been accused of being too abstract in their approach. Lupton (1999) argues that governmentality theorists devote too little attention to understanding how people respond to risk discourses and strategies. Like the Marxists they have attempted to better, they too are, perhaps, guilty of using brush strokes that are too broad and not painting in the detail of the picture they offer us. However, a number of the contributing authors of subsequent chapters within this book go some way towards addressing this deficiency by giving examples of how nurses and their clients adopt, negotiate and resist the risk discourses and strategies of health care within advanced liberalism.

Book chapters

In the Chapter 2 Andy Alaszewski offers an account of how risk was central to the development of health care institutions and in the transition to community, which gave rise to community nursing. He considers how community nursing is different from hospital-based nursing and how this difference affects community nurses' understanding of risk. Though community nurses have relatively more autonomy they are less able to control their working environment. Alaszewski examines how the varying conditions of different forms of community nursing are related to the ways in which community nurses understand and manage risk. After identifying a number of approaches and risk discourse within various areas of community practice, Alaszewski contrasts a narrow hazard approach with the advantages of a broad, negotiated and situated approach to risk.

In Chapter 3, Mary Ann Elston, Jonathan Gabe and Maria O'Beirne consider the issue of nurses being at risk of violence and aggression from patients and the public. Although research findings and statistical evidence indicate an increase in the incidence of violence against nurses, a changing understanding of what counts as violence or aggression, and changes in reporting practice may have produced this statistical increase. The authors examine recent UK policy initiatives in relation to violence. They suggest that calls for health workers to engage in formal risk assessment and to be zero-tolerant of even minor acts of aggression (bringing charges and regarding perpetrators of violence as criminals rather than patients) exemplify the themes of the govenmentality approach to risk.

Chapters 4 and 5 consider how risk discourse and practices are realised in mental health care nursing. In Chapter 4, it is argued that a particular type of 'risk thinking' has permeated and significantly changed mental health care policy and practices. The chapter explores Castel's thesis that the 'clinic of the subject' has transformed into the 'epidemiological clinic' and that danger has been converted into risk, to provide a detailed understanding of why and how 'risk thinking' has come to dominate mental health care and, more particularly, the work of mental health care nurses.

Chapter 5 offers an alternative understanding of how risk thinking may be understood within mental health care. Douglas's grid/group model is employed to develop a cultural understanding of how a forensic mental health care unit generates different perceptions, understandings and ways of dealing with risk amongst its staff and patients. Particular attention is given to differences between staff in different positions within the organisation and differences between the patients and the staff.

Chapter 6 provides an international component to the book. The authors, Karen MacKinnon and Liza McCoy, introduce us to the methodological and theoretical approach of Dorothy Smith to understanding risk. They examine the effects of Canadian preterm birth prevention programmes on the lives of pregnant women and families. MacKinnon and McCoy draw upon Smith's approach of 'institutional ethnography' to provide a feminist analysis of how risk discourses enter into the lives of childbearing women and nurses. Smith is strongly influenced by both Marx and Foucault. The value of her 'institutional ethnography' is to offer a way of providing detail to such abstract grand theory in the context of everyday life. In applying this approach MacKinnon and McCoy examine the work of nurses and other health care providers, in the Canadian context, to identify what Smith calls 'the conceptual practices of power' and how 'risk thinking' enters into institutional structures and nursing work processes.

Chapters 7, 8 and 9 all emphasise the dilemma of choice raised by the ongoing project within western society towards the elimination or, at least, minimisation of accidents, death, sickness and other undesirable events, through rational means. As the authors of these chapters illustrate, this project is highly problematic as the control of a multitude of risks will inevitably result in a multitude of consequences, thereby reducing some risks while increasing others. In Chapter 7, David Pontin explores the issues of risk and freedom for parents of children with life limiting and life threatening conditions and chronic health problems. Pontin draws from reflections and experiences of critical incidents in clinical practice to demonstrate how, for many parents, an important factor in the care they deliver to their children is managing the conflicting demands of the risks to their children's health against maintaining and providing a 'good' childhood. Pontin relates this project to the ideas of risk from Beck and Giddens, with concepts drawn from Bourdieu, and Fox to show how such social theory is relevant to the nursing of children with life limiting illnesses.

In Chapter 8, Bob Heyman and Jacqueline Davies explore the practices of caring for people with learning difficulties in a variety of multi-professional service contexts. Heyman and Davies suggest that the process of rehabilitation may be usefully understood in terms of clients being transformed from a position of confined safety towards greater personal autonomy. Particular attention is given to the competing values of service users, parents and professionals involved in this process and how risks are variously understood, prioritised and managed by each group.

In Chapter 9, Khim Horton considers how risk is balanced against independence in the nursing of older adults in a variety of care settings. This chapter considers the ways in which older people weigh social risks against perceived health risks to decide which is deemed the lesser of two evils. Horton then considers how the notion of 'trade-offs' is applied in caring for older people in the prevention of falls and how such nursing practices might be usefully re-examined and re-organised to balance risk aversion with social opportunity.

In Chapter 10, Anthony Pryce examines in detail the constructions of sexuality and sexual health risk and its management by the individual in contemporary society. In so doing Pryce employs a largely Foucauldian perspective, also informed by Douglas's ideas of purity and danger, and Gidddens's notion of reflexive modernity. Pryce argues that sexual categories and practices are being challenged and destabilised in contemporary society and that this contributes to increased risk of sexually acquired infections, giving rise to greater deployment of self-surveillance by the individual who must engage in ever more complex calculations of risk. Pryce suggests that there is ambivalence towards the erotic amongst health care professionals, some of whom construct sex and sexuality itself as a risk to the conduct of medical and nursing practice.

In Chapter 11, I attempt to offer some brief final thoughts about the theory and practice issues raised by all the contributing authors of the book. This might be particularly useful for those who loyally read the book from beginning to end. However, it is intended that the chapters of this book may be read independently from one another, so that readers who are interested in risk in relation to particular areas of nursing practice, might find what they are specifically looking for. The reader who is interested more generally in risk and nursing practice may be more inclined to read the entire book, though not necessarily in the order in which the chapters have been presented. I hope that this introductory chapter will serve as a useful outline of the main theoretical approaches to the sociology of risk as it can be applied to understanding nursing practice. I also hope that my brief outline of the content of the following chapters does justice to the book's contributing authors and inspires the reader to explore them all.

2 Managing risk in community practice: nursing, risk and decision-making

Andy Alaszewski

The development of modern nursing practice was closely linked to the development of health care institutions such as hospitals and asylums in the nineteenth century and its development outside such settings occurred more recently, mainly in the second half of the twentieth century. Since these two settings differ both in the type of risk which nurses are likely to experience and in the ways in which nurses assess and manage risk, I will compare and contrast these two settings before considering in more detail risk in community nursing practice.

Risk in institutional and community settings

Risk was central to the development of health care institutions and their internal structuring. A common theme in the history of institutions is the way in which they were established to manage dangers that threatened established order within society, whether such dangers came from infectious disease, crime, madness, vagrancy or degeneration of the population. Indeed, as Rothman noted in his study of the development of institutions in the United States of America, these threats were often seen as interlinked in the early nineteenth century, resulting in a common institutional response to a range of social issues (Rothman 1971).

Since institutions were designed to deal with risks, albeit risks associated with different types of hazard, they shared common physical and social structures and managed risk in similar ways. Risk was constructed and managed through the structuring of activities and relationships in time and space, through institutional routines and batch management of inmates or patients (see Goffman (1961) for a classic account of the 'total institution'). In acute hospitals, risks were primarily conceptualised in terms of biomedical threats, such as infection or contamination by pathogenic organisms or germs and controlled through institutional hygienic routines, for example, cleaning routines, asepsis and barrier nursing. This response is still evident in the ways in which hospitals and the government are responding to the 'superbug' Methicillin-Resistant Staphylococcus Aureus (MRSA). For example in England the Chief Nursing Officer at the Department of Health (DoH) launched a 'Think Clean Day' to raise the profile of good hygiene in hospitals to ensure safety (DoH 2005).

While these routines are overtly oriented towards the management of biomedical threats, they also have the effect of structuring relationships between nurses and patients enabling nurses to manage and process individuals through the system. Ethnographic studies of hospitals in the 1950s and 1960s clearly identified the ways in which these hygienic practices were used to structure space and manage or control the patients' passage through defined spaces and across prescribed boundaries. For example Rosengren and DeVault (1963) analysed the ways in which the physical structure of delivery suites was used to manage pregnancies. All women in labour passed through the same spaces and, by implication, stages of labour but at different speeds. Rapid deliveries were rushed through. Roth (1957) focused on the rituals which accompanied the control of risks. During work hours staff who entered potentially infected spaces wore protective clothing such as masks; outside work hours they entered the same space without taking protective measures against infection.

The major threats in acute hospital are depersonalised and externalised as 'germs' or 'superbugs'. However, in practice, individuals are a prime source of danger as carriers of, and the source of, infection. For example, in the Netherlands the response to MRSA has been to classify all patients and health-care workers who enter a hospital into one of four risk groups: Class A – proven, Class B – high risk, Class C – increased risk Class D – no risk (Vos 2005). Class A and B patients are nursed in islolation until they are shown to be safe. In England some hospitals have created security boundaries, preadmission clinics to screen patients to ensure that they are safe to be admitted (French 2005).

In psychiatric and learning disability institutions, there was no such externalisation, the hazard was located within and represented by each and every individual classified as mentally ill or learning disabled. In this context institutions were designed to identify and manage such risks and the threat they posed to wider society. The internal structure of the institution was not only a mechanism of control but also a mechanism for organising and displaying different forms of illness and disability. It was a taxonomy and a source of knowledge about the nature of illness and disability, the threat it posed and how such threats could and should be managed. This taxonomy was centred on risk. For example, Samuel Tuke, one of the main proponents in the early nineteenth century of Moral Treatment and institutional care for people with mental illness, stressed the importance of proper classification as the basis of effective treatment:

> Those who are violent, require to be separated from the more tranquil ... the patients are arranged into classes, as much as may be, according to the degree in which they approach rational or orderly conduct. (Tuke 1964 [1813]: 141)

The knowledge encoded in the taxonomy and the physical structure of the institution formed the basis of the identification and management of the risks associated with illness and disability. Key professionals, such as doctors, developed this structure through their scientific research and publication and, as Foucault (1971: 270) noted, had the standing and moral authority to apply it to individual cases through their expertise in diagnosing and prescribing treatment. This power involved not only control of institutional 'inmates' but also of the other institutional staff who managed inmates and the risks they presented on a day-to-day basis. In the early stages of the development of institutions these other staff were unskilled workers, in asylums, 'attendants', who were recruited and socialised into the institutional regime and its discourse.

With the development of professional education and training in the twentieth century, nursing played a more prominent role in assisting doctors in diagnosis and treatment, and in managing the day-to-day routine of the institutions, such as supervising nursing assistants or auxiliaries and student nurses. Thus, nurses occupied an important position within the staff hierarchy and the system of surveillance through which institutions identifed and managed risk. They had responsibilty for surveillance in a defined space, a unit or ward, over a period of time, a shift. They were responsible for observing, recording and reporting actions and activities of both patients and staff within this space, especially those who disrupted the routine and caused harm or threatened safety. In turn their actions were subject to surveillance both from senior nurses who had overall responsibility for the institution and by doctors who were responsible for care of the patients on the wards. Nurses, therefore, played a key role in the total institution which, by structuring space and time, sought to exercise the total surveillance of a panopticon, a system designed to make inmates permanently visible and observable (Foucault 1979: 201). This panopticon combined a physical structure with an asymetrical relationship between observer and observed and permitted

an internal, articulated and detailed control – to render visible those who were inside it ... the hospital building was gradually organized as an instrument of medical action: it was to allow better observation of patients, and therefore a better calibaration of their treatment; the form of the buildings, by careful separation of patients, was to prevent contagions. (Foucault, 1979: 172)

In reality institutions could not achieve the ideals of the panopticon. Design defects, lack of imaging technology such as CCTV and management problems meant that there were always spaces outside central surveillance and control. Within these spaces alternative cultures could and did develop, for example unit or ward level staff developed their own informal beliefs and practices (Belknap 1956) and inmates could exploit 'free places' outside the 'surveillance space' to sustain an underlife (Goffman 1961).

In the mid-twentieth century, there was a major shift in perceptions of risk and the associated responses to different forms of illness. Social and technological changes appeared to reduce the threat of illness while new treatments, especially drug therapies seemed to offer mechanisms for managing illness which were previously difficult to treat. For example, long-term improvements in diet and health plus new drug therapy meant that infectious diseases such as Tuberculosis (TB) were no longer major killers and such a threat to the health of the population (McKeown 1979). In mental health, and especially in learning disabilities, there was a shift in collective sensibility with a greater emphasis on the vulnerability of individuals rather than their dangerousness. New therapies such as psychoanalysis and drug therapies underpinned professional optimism that any elements of dangerousness could be effectively managed (Alaszewski 1983, 2003). These changes were linked to a major shift in the role of institutions within society. The role of institutions shifted from being the centre for managing all forms of risk to managing 'high' risk. Thus in acute hospitals, the emphasis in England was on district general hospitals to manage the acute high risk phases of illness requiring specialist expertise and technology. This meant that other hospitals such as local cottage hospitals, convalescence hospitals, longstay units for the chronically ill and specialist units for infectious disease such as TB sanatoria were surplus to requirements and low risk illness such as chronic illness could be managed in the community by GPs and community nurses. This shift was even more marked in the management of mental illness and learning disabilities. In mental illness it was accepted that there should be a role for institutions in the acute phase of illness but as a break with past practices and cultures these in-patient units were to be located within district general hospital structure. In learning disability, initially there was no role for institutions and all care was to be provided within community settings. In England and Wales these major changes in the role of institutions and the patterns of treatment and risk management were formally accepted as government policy in two white papers issued in the early 1960s on hospitals (Allen 1979, Ministry of Health (MoH) 1962) and community care (MoH 1963).

The precise implications of these changes for the nature of risk construction and management are the subject to debate. It is possible to argue that the development of care in the community did not in reality make a major difference in the management of risk. For example, Foucault argued that the development of psychoanalysis did not change the essential nature of power and control, and the need to manage the risk present in the patient; it merely shifted it from the structure of the institution to the practice of the doctor: 'To the doctor, Freud transferred all the structures Pinel and Tuke had set up in confinement' (Foucault 1971: 278). While the role of the institutions was considerably reduced, their influence over risk management in the community was maintained as they continued to manage the most dangerous patients and diseases. Heyman *et al.*, have conceptualised the overall system of care and risk management as a risk escalator which has three main characteristics:

> differentiation of steps in treatment regime in terms of the degrees of risk severity they are designed to manage; attempted congruence between varying levels of safety/autonomy balance and assessed client riskiness; and the potential to move individuals up towards increased safety (for self and/or others) and down towards greater autonomy. (Heyman *et al.* 2004: 310)

As Heyman *et al.*, note, such a model can be identified in a wide range of health care systems, for example, the system of screening babies to reduce the risk of their being born with chromosomal abnormalities, and to mental health and learning disabilities services, in which independent living represents the bottom of the escalator and forensic units the top.

Even if the institutional influence remains pervasive, it is important to recognise that there are significant differences between institutional and community settings that will shape the ways in which risk is identified and managed. Partly, this reflects the development of different groups of nurses working in the community. Mental health and learning disability nursing went through a process of deinstutionalisation with, in the case of learning disability, nursing a very strong and ideologically grounded rejection of institutional practice (Alaszewski and Ong 1990). In contrast, district nursing developed within the context of primary care. It also reflects major changes in the location of work. The institutional structure of classification, surveillance and control is significantly changed in the community. Much of the activity takes place within spaces that are not designed or controlled by professionals, for example, the service user's own home. While imaging technology can be installed within such spaces to observe, in practice, given limitation of resources, such technology is only installed in high risks environments, for example, in the homes of vulnerable individuals who are exposed to particular risks. In practice the activities of professionals within such spaces are virtually invisible to either their line managers or other professionals. Thus nurses working in the community are effectively operating in 'free places' outside surveillance. Such places are often controlled and managed by clients, and when entering them community nurses do not have the protection of the institutional environment and are of necessity forced to recognise and acknowledge the interest and concerns of the clients and therefore the ways in which clients define and manage risk. The practicalities of managing every-day interactions mean that community staff will develop their own routines of work. Lipsky (1980) argues that these routines make up a 'street-level bureaucracy' and one of their prime functions is to 'control clients and reduce the consequences of uncertainty' (1980: 86); in other words manage the risks of front-line work, and that such routines exist and function independently of agency policy which may or may not acknowledge and support them.

Nurses who work in the community are working on the frontline mostly outside the structure, protection and surveillance of the institution. There is pressure for them to effectively assess and manage risk, for example, a series of high profile inquiries in mental health services have highlighted public concerns and the need to identify and manage dangerous individuals (Ritchie Inquiry 1994). However, this does not necessarily mean that all nurses working in the community have internalised dominant definitions of risk. In the next section I will consider the extent to which nurses working in the community use definitions that challenge the dominant paradigm.

Defining risk: challenging dominant hazard-based definitions

As Eldridge and Hill (1999) have noted, an area of central importance in risk research is to explore which and whose definitions of risk are accepted in different contexts. While risk appears to have entered the English language during the seventeenth century its use and meaning have changed over time. Initially risk was associated with probability, especially with gambling and games of chance whose study created a specialist branch of mathematics, statistics (Douglas 1990). In modern society interest in risk has become more pervasive and linked to danger and the 'threat to desired outcomes' (Giddens 1991). However, risk is not only a way of managing the future but also serves a forensic function, the retrospective allocation of responsibility and blame when this process fails and significant harm, such as death, occurs (Douglas 1986: 59).

Contemporary health and welfare agencies are concerned with both aspects of risk, they need to identify risk so that they can avoid investigation and blame. In the mid-1990s my colleagues and I undertook a study of the risk policies of agencies and found that the operating definition of risk was risk as danger of hazard which had to be identified and managed to ensure the safety of service users (Alaszewski *et al.* 1998). Thus, one learning disability agency used hazard and harm interchangeably in its policy statement on identifying risk:

> The review should contain accurate information about the hazard, the risk, including evidence of the harm that can/has been caused by a particular risk. There is a strong argument for recording all risks then eliminating certain risks which are considered to be trivial ... immediate steps can be taken to eliminate risks where costs may be low and action simple. Merely to have reviewed will have raised a heightened awareness of risk. Actions should be recorded and taken. If some risk remains, the process will need to be continued. (Alaszewski *et al.* 1998: 55)

A starting point for reviewing the ways in which community nurses identify and manage risk, is to consider the ways in which they define risk and especially the congruence between their definitions of risk and the prominent 'risk as hazard' discourse. In another study, also in the 1990s, my colleagues and I looked at ways in which community nurses supporting vulnerable adults (including older people, people with mental health needs and people with learning disabilities) in the community, assessed and managed risk (Alaszewski *et al.* 2000). The research data that is used throughout the rest of this chapter has been drawn from both of these studies

Table 2.1 Definitions of risk

	Hazard	Balance	Opportunity
Mental health n = 24	21 (87.5%)	15 (62.5%)	5 (21%)
Older people n = 24	20 (83%)	16 (67%)	7 (29%)
Learning disability n = 24	18 (75%)	7 (29%)	10 (42%)
All nurses n = 72	59 (82%)	38 (53%)	22 (31%)

Note: Note in some interviews more than one definition was identified.

(see Table 2.1). In the second study, we started by examining the ways in which nurses conceptualised risk. While all the participants in our study, except for one group, accept that risk formed an important part of nursing practice and that risk tended to be an internalised taken-for-granted concept, when invited to define risk most nurses did not have an immediate response. They needed to pause to consider it and indeed some were initially reluctant to provide a definition. When they did articulate their reply, the majority (59, 82%) saw risk in terms of hazard and harm, especially the negative consequences of decisions or actions. For example, a community mental health nurse stated

> I see risk as a very negative thing because most of the risk that I'm dealing with is the risk of people self-harming or committing suicide

While a mental health nurse lecturer commented

> Risk to me connotes something negative, danger, needs something doing about it. It's dangerous, it's negative and something awful is going to happen.

Nurses using this approach did not need to justify or particularly elaborate on it as it fitted the dominant organisational approach to risk as they grouped together a whole range of issues. For example, one mental health nurse when asked whether he linked safety with risk, emphasised his managerial responsibility for a range of hazards:

> Yes, mainly around self-harm and harm to other people; but I think, again as a manager, being aware of legislation around health and safety at work, COSHH [Control of Substances Hazardous to Health] regulations, manual handling, those kinds of things and heightening staff awareness around those kinds of issues—infection control. We're having to get involved in both infection control and manual handling.

However, we also found definitions of risk that challenged the dominant risk paradigm. Nurses who recognised the possibility of alternative definitions of risk noted that this was a contested area and that the ways in which one definition had became prominent was the result of social processes not just the reflection of an objective reality. For example, a mental health nurse commented when invited to define risk.

That's the 50 million dollar question. What may be a risk for me may not be for another person – it very much depends on your point of view of what risk is. The definition causes me problems. The other thing I have a problem with is who has the right to define it because that will affect what you do about it.

Some nurses (22, 31%) argued for a more positive approach in which risk-taking was seen as a potentially liberating experience and an essential part of human growth and development. For example the learning disability nurses recognised that such an approach challenged the official or organisational definition to risk:

What I understand by risk and what the health authority understands is two different things. To me risk is a way of clients gaining knowledge, being able to develop, learn new things … often staff as well – the staff taking risks they actually learn things by that and learn what the clients can do from risks. The health authority thinks of risk as … protecting their backs.

While the risk as hazard approach can be seen as an internalisation of the dominant risk paradigm, discussions, which identified the positive aspects of risk, implied a degree of distrust of organisational motives, especially avoidance of bad publicity. Thus one mental health nurse described the impact of such publicity in the following way:

You only have to open the papers. I think this morning there was a sex offender escape from a medium secure unit. … As soon as anything like that happens, it has a knock-on effect for client decisions. … It depends politically what happens.

As a result nurses tended to justify this approach not by reference to organisational or even professional standards but by reference to the ordinariness of risk-taking as part of every-day life. For example a learning disability student nurse described risk in the following way:

> [It] depends on your point of view and style of life and philosophy. I might see going to the casino and gambling as a risk but someone else might not. [Risk can be defined as] a result of circumstances involving an activity. There is a risk in everything and it is what is 'acceptable'. Taking a gamble – the idea of being bad being more fun than being good. It's an aspect of life which most people enjoy – a bit of fear, getting the adrenaline going can be a good thing.

'Risk as a hazard to be identified and avoided' versus 'risk-taking as an opportunity for learning and development', represent two very different and apparently irreconcilable approaches. However, there was an intermediate position in which nurses (38, 58%) recognised both dangers and opportunities and saw risk as a process of balancing the two. A nurse with a community nursing background commented:

> [It's] part of allowing people to stay at home. If you've got older people living on their own it's that balance – it's the danger to themselves and the danger to the neighbour – it's when you start looking and say how far down the line can I go with these risks. But if someone is adamant, that they do not wish to move, in many ways it allows them to take that risk.

In this approach risk involves a recognition of hazard and danger but it also involves factoring in other aspects so that risk management is not restricted to hazard identification and management or safety at all costs, but involves identifying and balancing outcomes, safety versus autonomy. Adopting such an approach involves an element of trust. Accidents happen and on occasion users and others may be harmed. Nurses adopting this approach need to trust that the agency employing them will not hold them accountable and blame them if they can demonstrate that they acted reasonably.

Within all the areas of nursing within the community which we included in our study, the common sense approach of 'risk as a hazard to be identified and avoided' predominated. However, there was some variation between different groups of nurses. Mental health nurses tended to place the greatest emphasis on this approach. Learning disability nurses appeared more ready to recognise the positive aspects of risk taking while nurses providing support for older people were the most willing to recognise the balancing approach.

The mental health nurses in our study did acknowledge that their approach to risk emphasised the potential harmful consequences of the actions of acutely ill clients. They felt that this emphasis was a product of external pressure on nurses in this area of practice. In particular they were concerned about the potential consequences of high-profile incidents in which acutely ill individuals had harmed themselves, members of the public or individuals providing them with support. Such incidents had resulted in public inquires which had attracted considerable media coverage and resulted in the allocation of blame. As Cambridge has noted such inquiries 'seek to allocate some level of individual responsibility or blame' (2004: 235). For example, the committee of inquiry into the killing of Jonathan Zito by Christopher Clunis (Ritchie Inquiry 1994) highlighted the failure of individual practitioners to effectively assess the danger posed by Christopher Clunis. It recommended that in the case of patients who had been violent, aftercare plans should include 'an assessment ... as to whether the patient's propensity for violence presents any risk to his own health or safety, or to the protection of the public' (Ritchie Inquiry 1994: 111). Mental health nurses in our study saw a link between high-profile media coverage and a narrow defensive approach to risk. One mental health nurse articulated this link in the following way:

> *Interviewer:* 'What's happening that's made people more aware [of risk]?'
>
> *Nurse A:* 'It's probably because there's less hospital beds and closing down of institutions.'
>
> *Nurse B:* 'High media profile'.
>
> *Nurse A:* 'And ever since Ben Sillcott[1] ... just jumped into the lion's den it's become a very hot topic ... So a lot of it's to do with media coverage ... and that has made management more aware and that filters down to clinicians' level

Mental health nurses in our study felt that there was pressure from Government ministers and the Department of Health to prevent such incidents and to ensure that professionals identified and managed hazards effectively.

---

[1] Ben Sillcott was a young man diagnosed as suffering from schizophrenia who became famous as a failure of community care when he decided to cross safety barriers to enter the lion enclosure in London Zoo.

Risk and decision making

While definitions provide some indication of the ways in which nurses structure risk, these definitions are an indirect measure of the actual risk management practices; there can be a significant gap between saying and doing. Examining the ways in which community nurses make decisions about users is one way of exploring actual practices. As Narayan and Corcoran-Perry have noted 'Decision-making tasks of interest in professional domains are characterised by complexity, ambiguity, and uncertainty' (1997: 354).

We invited 20 community nurses to record their decision-making in a clinical log or diary (see Table 2.2). Through this process we identified 584 separate decisions. Most of these (464, 80%) involved client care. We also identified decisions that concerned the nurses' own situation, especially work load or safety issues; for example, one experienced district nurse recorded her decision to question workloads and activities:

> Meeting at 12 with our Team Manager. We are told that the over 75s service is to be within our remit. [I] advised the manager we have trouble getting reassessments done. Apparently she wasn't aware! It is clear that she doesn't fully understand our role as District Nurses and seems to relate to hospital nurses. [I] had to put forward what we see as our role as, and that we just do not go into homes and fill in forms without looking at the patient as a whole. This is taking our accountability to the full, rather than creating face to face contact [to fulfil the conditions of the] GP contract.

We explored and examined the decision-making process, in particular identifying whether nurses used structured decision making, negotiating methods or intuition. Structured decision making can be linked to a hazard approach as it involves checklists to assess risk and guidelines for making decisions and leaves an audit trail that can be used to demonstrate that

Table 2.2 The process of decision making (20 diarists)

	Formal %	Negotiated %	Intuition %
Mental health nurses n = 160	31	48	21
Community nurses n = 274	45	22	33
Learning disability nurses n = 113	19	39	42
All nurses n = 584	35	33	32

reasonable efforts were made to identify and account for risk. Negotiation can be linked to a definition of risk which recognises the existence of different and conflicting definitions of risk and therefore, by implication, the need through negotiation, to create the best possible balance and, where possible, maximise support for a decision. Intuition can be linked to the risk-taking approach as it emphasises personal empathy and the use of every-day common sense.

The differences between such approaches can be seen in the diary entries. In the following extract, an experienced district nurse describes how she responded to a serious incident, which could have had fatal consequences; a client, without realising, burnt her legs on a gas fire:

> Outlined risk of gas fire [to client] + advised not to sit directly in front of fire + keep legs away from direct heat. Assessed other aspects of safety – seemed to be no other problems. Water low – low risk Lifting + handling – no risk. Social services involved = has home help. Visits organised for 3x weekly.

An experienced community psychiatric nurse (CPN) also recorded her use of structured approach to justify her decisions not to accept three referrals for further treatment:

> a.m. CPN Clinic three referrals – Reasons for referral two stress reaction and one grief reaction. Each referral received one hour assessment. Decision made not to offer further appointment, assessment also encompassed 'risk'. CPN clinic used as a 'screening' to facilitate decision to accept client into Mental Health [services]. I believe my training is sufficient to formulate decision regarding option of accepting or declining referral. My decision is based upon Generic Psychiatric Assessment–Risk Assessment and Research based practice stating reactive mental health resolves its problem without CPN involvement, affectionately known as the 'worried well'.

The nurse in this situation was able to use a structured approach to her decision as the nature of the decision was relatively easy to define, namely whether or not to accept the patients into the service, she could identify specific methods of identifying information and she felt there was a structured evidence base that she could draw on to justify her decision. However, in many situations the nature of the decision is complex, there are competing interests and no amount of additional evidence will assist in the process. In such contexts negotiation is often used. For example the following decisions involved an experienced district nurse who felt that she was under pressure to increase the dosage of a painkiller to dangerous levels and reached an agreement with the patient's GP to maintain the current dosage:

31st March

Terminal lady on syringe driver [for pain relief]. One colleague, who worked over the weekend has suggested that the Diamorphine need[ed] to be increased. On visit this morning and pm I felt this was not justified. Family not in attendance and the manager of the home agree[d] with me in one way but also remark[ed] that the family had taken 3 days off work [in anticipation of patients death]!! I need to review this lady condition in the morning to feel that the increase is justified for the patient rather than the family/home. Being a patient advocate is not easy, or black and white when a situation like this occurs. I am aware what the increase will do but I also see that the patient is very comfortable and not in pain.

1st April

Early start with patients before meeting the GPs at 8.30am. Needed to discuss with GP re the syringe driver [who agrees to maintain dose] ... Reference the syringe driver. The family still seem unhappy, even with the GP decision, of maintain[ing] the Diamorphine dose. I feel this was the right decision I now have to discuss this with the family and advise referral to GP if they want to do so. Handling relatives with this issue cannot be given in training. Even with a broad amount of training in bereavement will not prepare how either you will react or the relatives in a given situation. Maybe scenarios or role play may help.

In the diaries we were also able to identify decisions based on intuition which were grounded in the personal knowledge and expertise that the nurse has developed over time, for example knowledge of specific clients. Nurses could use such knowledge to identify 'warning signals' by attaching specific meaning and significance to relatively minor comments or actions. For example in the following diary extract, an experienced CPN indicated how he used his personal knowledge of a client to identify warning signals and prioritise a particular case to prevent a potential suicide:

Message on answerphone from Client M. She wants to talk to me. When I phone back she says she doesn't need me, she is going to [famous landmark on the English coast]. As she is not driving at the moment, I question this and she hangs up. M. was previously admitted to hospital before Easter when I prevented her from taking herself to the sea 'to join her sister' who had been dead for a number of years. My decision is to cancel my first client and go round to M. I find her staring through the window, refusing to let me in. Eventually I persuade her to open the door. She is monosyllabic, apparently attending to and responding to voices. She then indicated to me that she is going to drive off [famous landmark on the English coast] to join her sister. I arrange for the ward to take her ... and she is admitted.

While there is clearly pressure for nurses to adopt a hazard-based approach to risk management and to use structured systems to assess and manage risk, nurses in our study felt able to resist such pressures when appropriate. Overall there was a relatively even division between the different approaches to decision making and risk with a small preponderance of formal decision making and less evidence of intuitive decision making. However, there were important differences between the various areas of nursing. Community nurses emphasised formal decision making reflecting the development of risk assessment tools, such as those used to assess pressure sores, plus evidence-based guidelines. Nevertheless, they were also willing and able to use intuition; indeed some nurses stressed the need for different forms of knowledge as in the following extract from the diary of an experienced district nurse:

> Training gave me knowledge and awareness of risk, and tools used not only became part of every day working with experience and practice in the community and drawing on past experience.

Learning disability nurses made the most use of intuition and also engaged in negotiation. Mental health nurses appeared to be less willing than other nurses to take the personal responsibility implicit in the use of intuition and keener to share responsibility or to ground their decisions in a formal structured approach.

Conclusion

When professionals assess and treat individuals they utilise skills based on knowledge. Professionals can use different types of knowledge which they acquire from different sources. For example, evidence-based practice is based on knowledge acquired from the systematic evaluation of practice. This type of knowledge can be referred to as encoded knowledge (Lam 2000) as it is often collected and codified in documents such as clinical guidelines. In contrast reflective practice is based on knowledge acquired by an individual practitioner and based on reflection of individual cases (Benner 1984; Schön 1988). It can be classified as embodied knowledge as it is used intuitively by individual professionals to respond to the unique circumstances of a particular case. Lam (2000) identifies two other forms of knowledge, 'embrained' which is based on an individual's use of cognitive and conceptual skills to solve problems, and 'embedded' which is based on the development of shared routines that have been successful in the past. Current pressure in risk assessment and management involves an emphasis on encoded knowledge:

> Medicine combines aspects of both 'embrained' and 'embodied' knowledge, and ... current schemes of clinical governance represent a drive to transform medicine into 'encoded knowledge' (especially through the promulgation of Clinical Guidelines by NICE ...). (Flynn 2002: 168)

Such changes will reduce the individual scope of professional autonomy and judgement. However, at present, there is little evidence to indicate whether the changes will improve the quality of decision making and the safety of users.

While Beck (1992) has characterised contemporary society as Risk Society, increasingly health and welfare agencies can be seen as Risk or Safety Agencies. As Kemshall has argued

> Risk, particularly an individualized and responsibilized risk, is replacing need as the core principle of social policy formation and welfare delivery. (Kemshall 2002: 1)

Kemshall analysed the ways in which the development of more responsive public services which are 'safety oriented' is reshaping public services. A more responsive public service is not only more exposed to risk as it is expected to reach higher standards, often on lower resources, but is also subject to greater scrutiny through audit systems which are often linked to naming and shaming mechanisms. As Kemshall has noted the culture of safety as evidenced in various health and social care inquiries has been a major factor in this development:

> Our era is dominated by a peculiarly defensive attitude to risk, which Frank Furedi ... has labelled a 'culture of safety' in which risks are almost always framed by the precautionary principle of 'better safe than sorry'. (Kemshall 2002: 1)

Thus central to the current restructuring of public services is replacement of need as the key principle of welfare rationing and provision, the observation with risk and vulnerability. In some services, such as child protection, mental health and probation services, this process is quite advanced (Kemshall 1998, 2002). An important issue is whether this change will bring benefits and if so for whom. This depends how risk is defined and used (Kemshall 2000). If risk is defined in a narrow hazard-orientated way then risk management can be a mechanism of protecting the agency and its employees from blame and litigation at the cost of restricting users' choices and rights. If, on the other hand, it is defined in a broader more creative way, for example, as reasonable risk-taking, then it can be used as a way of empowering service users. Given current pressures on agencies and the professionals they employ, from Inquiries, the Government and the media, it seems likely that there will be continued pressure for nurses working within the community to adopt a structured approach to decision making which emphasises the importance of systematically identifying and counteracting hazards.

3 A 'risk of the job'? violence against nurses from patients and the public as an emerging policy issue

Mary Ann Elston, Jonathan Gabe and Maria O'Beirne

Introduction

'Why are nurses more at risk than these bouncers?' was the striking headline (accompanied by photographs of muscle-bound men) carried by one of many features on violence against nurses in the *Nursing Times* (NT) over the past decade (Coombes 1999: 17). A recent critical account of the state of nursing in Britain goes further: 'Nursing is now arguably the most dangerous job in Britain', and the context for this claim is specifically work-related violence (Hart 2004: 255, 263–265). The published research literature on violence against nurses has increased sharply since the 1980s (Poster and Ryan 1993; Wells and Bowers 2002). A recent systematic review of the international research literature on the non-somatic effects of violence on nurses identified more than 6600 items published between 1983 and 2003 in its initial search (Needham *et al.* 2005).

In the United Kingdom (UK),[1] research on violence against health workers in various settings has been commissioned by both government and professional organisations (for example, Gournay 2002, United Kingdom Central Council for Nursing

---

[1] Strictly speaking, most of the material in this paper, particularly the discussion of policy, relates specifically to the NHS in England but the general themes are equally relevant to other parts of the UK.

(UKCC) 2002 and Wright *et al.* 2002). Such bodies have also actively promulgated policy initiatives, research dissemination conferences and guidance for preventing and managing work-related violence in health care (for example, Health Services Advisory Committee 1997, Royal College of Nursing (RCN) 1998 and NMC (Nursing and Midwifery Council 2004). A recent development was the publication, in 2005, of the National Institute for Clinical Excellence (NICE) guideline *Violence: the short-term management of disturbed/violent behaviour in psychiatric in-patient and emergency settings* (NICE 2005). In 2004, the National Health Service (NHS) in England announced plans for what has been claimed to be the largest ever training programme in the United Kingdom (UK), if not in Europe, a one day 'conflict resolution course' to be made available to all front-line NHS staff: potentially 730,000 people (Oxtoby 2004). This training programme is a continuation of earlier government initiatives, particularly the cross-government 'NHS Zero Tolerance Zone' (ZTZ) campaign launched in 1999. The ZTZ campaign aimed to raise awareness among staff of the need to report violent incidents to their managers and of the action that might be taken against perpetrators, and required NHS trusts to develop local prevention and reduction strategies. Its key message to NHS staff and to the public was that violence and intimidation should no longer be tolerated as an inevitable 'risk of the job'. 'We don't have to take this' is the recurrent ZTZ slogan (Department of Health (DoH) 1999b and c). In total, including successive relaunches of the ZTZ campaign, the Department of Health (DoH) announced at least 14 'key initiatives aimed at reducing and ultimately preventing violence and aggression against NHS staff' between 1997 and 2002 (National Audit Office 2003b: 41).

In sum, although it is frequently re-iterated that violence against nurses (or health care workers as a whole) is not a new phenomenon, it has recently been 'rediscovered' as a significant, and, according to many, a growing problem (Paterson and Leadbetter 1999). Work-related violence is now identified as a major financial as well as human risk facing the NHS. In 2003, the National Audit Office (NAO) (the body responsible for scrutinising public expenditure on behalf of Parliament) suggested, as a 'crude estimate,' that the direct cost of violence to the NHS was at least £69 million per annum. This estimate excludes costs of staff replacement and treatment and compensation, and takes 'no account of the human costs, such as physical and/psychological pain and increased stress levels, which are known to be substantial, nor the impact of violence and aggression on staff confidence and retention' (NAO 2003b: 4). The NAO estimated that violent incidents represented 40 per cent of all recorded health and safety incidents in the NHS and concluded that, 'Although all staff are vulnerable, nurses experience the highest numbers of incidents' (NAO 2003b: 9).

In this chapter, we provide an analysis of this (re-)emergent policy and professional concern with violence as one of the risks of nursing work. In undertaking our analysis, we find ourselves treading a difficult line. On the one hand, there is much evidence that nurses in the UK do face a relatively high risk of work-related violence compared with most other occupations. This evidence and every individual attack on a nurse are clearly matters for concern. At the same time, it is important to subject the evidence, claims about the risk and associated policy measures to critical scrutiny. This is what we aim to do in this chapter, focusing on policy and managerial issues, rather than on how nurses themselves, individually and collectively, experience and manage violence. At the risk of underplaying the heterogeneity of nursing and health care settings, much of the analysis in this short chapter is fairly general. This reflects the way in which work-related violence has increasingly been framed as a risk for all nurses or, indeed, for all health workers, not just those working in settings long regarded as carrying relatively high risk, such as acute in-patient psychiatric wards (Noble and Rodger 1989).

In focusing only on violence *from* service users and the public *to* nurses, we do not intend to imply that violence between health care workers never occurs;[2] nor that responsibility for violence involving service users rests always with the public or

---

[2] At least in the nursing literature, work-based conflict between nurses, so-called 'horizontal violence', is often analysed in terms of nursing being an oppressed and subordinated occupation, rather than in terms of occupational risk (e.g.,

patients; nor that the distinction between perpetrators and victims of violence is always clear. Cases in which nurses have been deemed to be at fault are part of the complex context for both policy and practice in managing violence to nurses. One high profile recent case was that of David 'Rocky' Bennett, a patient who, in 1998, died in an NHS psychiatric secure unit as a result of being forcibly pinioned to the floor after he had assaulted a nurse. According to the official inquiry that eventually took place, inappropriate use of restraint by nurses followed a history of substandard and racist treatment of Mr Bennett (Gould 2004).

Finding the appropriate balance between protecting both staff and the public and therapeutic management, and between best practice in risk management and professional obligations to each individual patient, pose recurrent dilemmas for policymakers, health care providing organisations, and individual health care workers in their daily practice (UKCC 2002). In this chapter we show how the emerging issue of work-related violence has come to be framed in terms of risk assessment and management. We begin with the problem of identifying and measuring risk, with the definition of violence.

Definitions of violence: finding a rational basis for calculating risk?

In current policy and social research literature on violence in general, considerable attention is devoted to the definition of violence, discussing what the term means to relevant actors, and how it should be operationalised in research and in organisational records. Thus, one key thread running through the recent social research literature on this topic is that what counts as violence varies over time and according to social context: and that the meaning of the term is sometimes contested.

Farrell, G. A. (2001) 'From tall poppies to squashed weeds: why don't nurses pull together more?' *Journal of Advanced Nursing*, 35, 1, 26–33, Freshwater, D. (2000) 'Crosscurrents: against cultural narration in nursing', *Journal of Advanced Nursing*, 32, 2, 481–484, Roberts, S. J. (1983) 'Oppressed group behaviour: implications for nursing', *Advances in Nursing Science*, 5, July, 21–30.

For example, in their review of social research on violence in organisations, Hearn and Parkin (2001) identify three possible definitions. First, 'violence' can be equated with *physical violence*, or even specifically with physical assaults involving injury. This definition, by implication, draws a distinction between violence and non-physical forms of transgressive behaviour such as verbal abuse, harassment or bullying. A second possibility Hearn and Parkin identify is to use an expanded definition that includes such behaviour as harassment and bullying, even when these take such forms as slander and gossip, or jeering. A third option (favoured by Hearn and Parkin) 'is to adopt a broad, socially contextualised understanding of violence as violation ... violence [is] those structures, actions, events and experiences that violate, cause violation or are considered as violating. ... Violence can thus ... include intimidation, interrogation, surveillance, persecution, subjugation, discrimination and exclusion that lead to experiences of violation' (Hearn and Parkin 2001: 18).

The first definition is the one conventionally associated with the criminal law and has, historically, underpinned many official recording systems. The use of physical force (and the extent of any resulting injury) are important considerations in determining whether and what criminal charges might be brought against an alleged offender and how employers should respond to incidents. In the UK, there is a specific statutory requirement for employers to report, to the Health and Safety Executive, any physical assaults and other accidents that result in physical injuries necessitating employees being off work for three days or more (RIDDOR (Reporting of Injuries) 1995). However, since the 1970s, this relatively restrictive definition, of violence as physical force, has been extensively criticised for its focus on what some regard as only one among many types of violence. In particular, feminist campaigners and researchers in the field of sexual violence have argued that emphasising physical assault and injury risks obscuring or trivialising, for example, verbal abuse, sexual harassment or intimidation, and the emotional and psychological consequences of aggressive acts, whether or not physical injury is incurred (see Kelly and Radford 1996). As a result of such criticisms, there has been a shift in social science research on violence towards using wider definitions similar to the second or even the third approach identified by Hearn and Parkin. In the process, attention has moved somewhat away from the acts and the intentions of the perpetrators to the 'victims' and the risk, in the broadest sense, for 'victims' and for society. The same shift towards an inclusive definition of violence is also detectable in many policy sectors. Here great emphasis is placed on the importance of agencies using standardised definitions in order to render violence a rationally calculable risk, so as to provide the basis for prevention and management strategies. For example, in relation to work-related violence, the European Commission has adopted the following inclusive definition:

[Work-related] violence means any incident where staff are abused, threatened or assaulted in circumstances related to their work, involving an explicit or implicit challenge to their safety, well-being or health. (Wynne *et al.* 1997)

This is the definition formally adopted by the NHS Executive in the ZTZ campaign, and which all NHS organisations and their staff are expected to follow in recording incidents of violence. Thus, the current official definition of violence in the NHS emphasises the impact of violence on staff and includes much more than physical assaults, as shown below in Table 3.1. The dominant message of ZTZ to NHS staff is that they 'don't have to take' any of these behaviours, whatever the state of physical or mental health of perpetrators. Thus the ZTZ definition recognises that, for example, being subjected to abusive or threatening phone calls from a patient's relative might have as much or more impact on a nurse's 'well-being or health' than being scratched by a very elderly, confused patient, but regards both incidents as violence which ought to be reported to the management. In the rest of this chapter we use the term 'violence' inclusively, according to the ZTZ definition, unless otherwise indicated, distinguishing where appropriate between different forms of violence.

This inclusive definition of violence, however, is by no means universally used by NHS and other health care organisations or in current research. For example, in the

Table 3.1 What constitutes workplace violence?

Physical violence	Non-physical violence
• Assault causing death	• Verbal abuse, swearing or shouting, name calling and insults
• Assault causing serious physical injury (requiring hospital treatment)	• Racial or sexual harassment
• Minor injuries requiring first-aid	• Threats – with or without weapons
• Physical attack not causing injury (kicking, biting, punching)	• Physical posturing and/or threatening gestures
• Use of weapons and/or missiles	• Abusive telephone calls or letters
• Sexual assault	• Bullying
	• Deliberate silence

Source: National Audit Office (NAO) 2003b: 46.

research on violence in acute in-patient mental health care commissioned by the UKCC, the term 'violence' is specifically identified with physical force, as distinct from 'abuse' or 'aggression' (Wright *et al.* 2002).[3] The recently issued NICE guideline relating to the same clinical area also follows this definition (NICE 2005: 82).

Of course, drawing a terminological distinction between violence and, for example, verbal abuse, does not necessarily imply that the latter is regarded as trivial. For example, in 2004, the *NT* launched a campaign to 'Rule out Abuse', with an editorial that declared, 'Violence towards health professionals is highly visible and well documented, yet verbal abuse remains a problem with a low profile'. The editorial was accompanied by the report of a *NT* readers' survey, which found that approximately nine in ten respondents had been verbally abused at work at some time in their career (Anonymous 2004; Norris 2004). Nor does using the term 'violence'

---

[3] In the UKCC commissioned research, '*Violence* refers to the use of physical force which is intended to hurt or injure another person. *Aggression* refers to a disposition, a willingness to inflict harm, regardless of whether this is behaviourally expressed and physical harm is sustained. *Verbal aggression* refers to verbal abuse or threats' (Wright *et al.* 2002: 7).

inclusively preclude drawing distinctions between sub-types of violence, as when the ZTZ campaign launched a specific initiative on harassment (NHS Executive 2002). Indeed, we would argue that being able to make such distinctions in data may often be very important, for example, in understanding the meaning of different types of incident to 'victims'.[4]

Our purpose in drawing attention to inconsistencies between and contestation over definitions of violence is, first, to alert readers to the difficulties in practice of comparing different sources of data on 'violence', notwithstanding the emphasis in recent policy guidance on developing standardised definitions for research and organisational monitoring. But, second, we wish to draw out further implications of moving to a more inclusive definition. It is almost axiomatic that the more inclusive the definition of 'violence' employed, the greater will be the reported prevalence rate of untoward incidents. Verbal abuse, for example, is almost certainly more frequently experienced than physical assault in nursing work. So, to take as an example the *NT* survey quoted earlier, if respondents were representative of nursing as a whole, virtually all nurses should expect to have at least one episode of verbal abuse, that is, of violence according to the ZTZ definition, in a nursing career. Thus, violence comes to be established as a very frequent, statistically normal experience for nurses.

Seeking recognition that violence was a frequent experience at least for women was an important impetus behind feminist calls for more inclusive definitions of violence from the 1970s (Kelly and Radford 1996). By expanding the range of behaviours

---

[4] Our approach in our own empirical research was to use specific terms such as 'physical assault', 'threat' and 'verbal abuse', in questionnaires without prejudging which of these should be regarded as 'violence'. We also sought to ascertain, through in-depth interviews, the meaning of the term 'violence' to different occupational groups. (See Gabe, J., Denney, D., Lee, R. M., Elston, M. A., and O'Beirne, M. (2001) 'Researching professional discourse on violence', *British Journal of Criminology*, 41, 3, 460–471. O'Beirne, M., Denney, D., Gabe, J., Elston, M. A., and Lee, R. M. (2003). Veiling violence: the impacts of professional and personal identities on the disclosure of work-related violence. In Lee, R. M. and Stanko, E. A. (eds.), *Researching Violence: Essays on Methodology and Measurement* (pp. 177–191). London: Routledge.)

to be labelled as 'violence', women's experience of sexual harassment, intimidation and domestic abuse was rendered more visible and more clearly unacceptable to women themselves and, gradually, to institutions such as the police, rather than being dismissed as either trivial or women's inevitable fate. For example, some feminists argued that, rather than regarding rape as the action of a highly deviant minority of evil or psychologically disturbed individuals, and verbal sexual harassment as normal male behaviour to be tolerated, both should be regarded as points on a single continuum of (sexual) violence. And, it was argued, all sexual violence was to be regarded as primarily a means by which men in general exercised power over women, see Stanko (1996).[5]

Of course, those who recommend an inclusive definition of violence in other contexts, such as the workplace, may not consciously adhere to an explanatory model which regards violence as an expression of power. But, as indicated above, expanding the range of behaviours to be counted as work-related violence may not only render 'violence' as being a relatively normal experience for nurses. It also increases the number of persons who are to be counted as perpetrators of violence, changing them from members of a rare, deviant minority to potentially any patient or member of the public. The point is that the drive to adopt inclusive definitions of violence has been partly underpinned by a very different understanding of violence from one that sees patients' violence as a consequence of their health problems. Perhaps it is not a coincidence that it is in the context of acute mental health care that the restrictive definition of violence as physical assault and a medicalised explanatory model appear to prevail. Later in the paper we return to the implications of these different models of violence and of the violent. Before doing so we review some recent evidence about the scale of violence against nurses in the UK.

---

[5] An extreme form of this was the claim, in the 1970s, by prominent radical American feminist Susan Brownmiller that 'all men are rapists', and that rape is a 'process of intimidation by which all men keep women in a state of fear' Brownmiller, S. (1976) *Against Our Will*. Harmondsworth: Penguin.

Measuring risk: assessing the prevalence of violence

Given the variations in definition described above, it will be apparent that the proliferating statistical evidence on the prevalence of violence to UK health care staff needs to be approached with caution (see Committee of Public Accounts 2003, Lee and Stanko 2003, Wells and Bowers 2002). There are two main types of data source on work-related violence – organisational records and victim surveys. In the case of organisational records, it has been widely accepted that many incidents of violence and aggression at work go unrecorded, even when there are established reporting procedures and definitions within the organisation. Nursing is not likely to be an exception here, although there is evidence that doctors are particularly reluctant to report health and safety incidents (NAO 2003b: 18). One study of a psychiatric in-patient setting compared videotape evidence with incident reports, revealing 155 videotaped assaults (not all by patients on staff) compared to 12 officially recorded incidents over the study period (Crowner *et al.* 1994). In health care, under-reporting may arise for many reasons, including the dismissal of incidents as trivial (although not all serious incidents are reported), or discountable because of patients' medical conditions. Staff may perceive reporting procedures as too cumbersome or consider that making a report would bring little benefit and might possibly disadvantage them; for example, stigma from apparent failure of professional competence or the initiation of further time-consuming procedures (Beale 1999; Cembrowicz and Shepherd 1992).

It follows that changes in reporting practices can produce artefactual changes in recorded rates of work-related violence. This appears to have happened in the NHS since the inception of the ZTZ programme. The ZTZ programme aimed to improve management systems for reporting and recording violence within NHS organisations, including universal adoption of the inclusive ZTZ definition, and to increase the use of such systems by staff. Even partial achievement of these aims would be likely bring about an increase in recorded incidents of violence. So, it is not very surprising that officially recorded incidents of violence against NHS trust staff in England have risen from approximately 65,000 in 1998–1999 (before the ZTZ campaign was fully underway) to almost 84,000 in 2001/2002 and 95,000 in 2002/2003 (an increase of 46 per cent in five years).

In 2003, the NAO attributed much of the increase in officially recorded incidents to 'better awareness of reporting with more widespread use of the common [ZTZ] definition which includes verbal abuse'. Although noting that 'increased hospital activity, higher patient expectations and frustrations due to increased waiting times' might be factors, the NAO concluded that, with respect to violence in NHS trusts:

> Wide variations in reporting standards, different definitions and con-
> tinued under-reporting, make it impossible to say conclusively how far
> the increase in reported violence reflects an actual increase in inci-
> dents or measure how trusts, individually or overall, are performing.
> There also remains a high and varied level of under-reporting of inci-
> dents (which we estimate is around 39 per cent). (NAO 2003b: 2)

The other main type of data source is the 'victim' survey: retrospective data collection, usually by structured question-naire, about the experience of violence from relevant samples. In general, these tend to show higher prevalence rates (the chances of individuals' having been a victim over a specified time period) than organisational records for comparable work settings. But comparison between different surveys is often difficult because of variations in operationalising and measur-ing violence and sampling variations. One problem with many surveys specifically about work-related violence is the likely response bias. Those who have experienced work-related vio-lence may be more likely to respond than those who have not, leading to over-estimates of risk, even where the original sam-ple was representative of the target population. Surveys like that from the *NT* cited above, should be treated with special caution because of this, and because *NT* readers may not be representative of the nursing profession as a whole, with respect to the work they do and the work-related violence they encounter.

One of the most respected sources of survey data on work-related violence in the UK is the British Crime Survey (BCS), a Home Office-funded survey of a large, nationally representative sample (c.36,000 respondents in 2002/2003), conducted regularly since 1991 (Budd 1999, 2001; Upson 2004). With a response rate of over 70 per cent and questions about many forms of crime victimisation besides violence at work, the BCS is probably not subject to the particular response bias noted above. But its definition of violence is more restrictive than, for example, that used in the ZTZ campaign. Reflecting its orientation to criminal offences, the BCS's questions about violence at work relate only to 'all assaults or threats which occurred while the victim was working and were perpetrated by members of the public', and not, for example, to verbal abuse (Budd 2001: 2).

In contrast to the widespread view that work-related violence is currently on the increase, the general trend identified by the BCS is that the overall risk for all workers of being assaulted has fallen by 32 per cent from a peak in 1997 to levels in 2002/2003 (the latest year for which figures are available) that are slightly below those in 1991 when the BCS began. However, the BCS does clearly indicate, as do many other surveys comparing different occupations (e.g., International Labour Organisation *et al.* 2002, Wells and Bowers 2002) that the chance of being a victim of assaults and threats at work (the prevalence rate) is higher for health workers than for most occupations and, among qualified health workers, highest for nurses. However, the prevalence rate for qualified nurses has been consistently less than that for protective service workers (police, fire service, prison service). The rate for qualified nurses has remained fairly constant since the mid-1990s, with approximately 5 per cent of qualified nurses reporting being either assaulted or threatened at work in the previous 12 months (Budd 1999, 2001; Upson 2004).[6]

---

[6] In the 2002/2003 BCS report, qualified nurses were included in a category 'health and welfare associate professionals', which includes midwives, professions allied to medicine and some welfare workers. However, as nurses are by far the largest occupation within this category, the figures may be broadly comparable to previous years. (Nursing assistants and nurse managers are included in other occupational categories.) It is not possible to distinguish between different nursing fields (or identify prevalence rates specifically for nightclub 'bouncers') in the published BCS reports, Upson, A. (2004) *Violence at Work: Findings from the 2002/2003 British Crime Survey: Home Office Online Report 04/04.* London: Home Office.

This prevalence rate is lower than those found in two other recent national surveys, probably because of differences in sampling and in the definition of violence. The nurses in the BCS's sample may be in any field of nursing, in or outside the NHS, and affiliated to any professional or trade union organisation or none. In contrast, the RCN's *Working Well* survey in 2002 was of a random sample of 6000 of its full members (In total 4100 questionnaires were returned, a response rate of 68.5 per cent). This survey covered a range of topics related to nurses' health and well-being, including violence, and found that 34 per cent of all respondents had been 'harassed or assaulted' by a patient or patient's relative in the past 12 months (only half of whom had completed an accident form following an incident). Overall, 30 per cent of these RCN respondents reported having been physically assaulted at some time in their careers (RCN 2002).

A second, relatively new source of national data is what is intended to be a regular annual survey the NHS National Staff Survey (NSS) first conducted in 2003 by the Commission for Health Improvement, now superseded by the Healthcare Commission. In 2003 and 2004 the main NSS covered staff employed by the 572 NHS trusts in England providing acute/specialist, ambulance, mental health and primary care services. Bank and agency staff and GPs and their directly employed staff are not included, but all trust-employed non-clinical staff, including managers, clerical and technical staff are. In 2004, questionnaires were sent to over 360,000 staff, with 60 per cent responding. Overall, the 2004 NSS found that a significant number of respondents had experienced physical violence or some form of bullying, non-physical abuse or harassment from patients or their relatives during the previous 12 months. The report provides a detailed break down of this response – analysing the difference between trusts, and between doctors, registered nurses and health care assistants. Unfortunately, we were not granted permission to include more detailed analysis of the surveys in this chapter, but data on occupational groups, can be found online at: http://www.healthcarecommission.org.uk/ NationalFindings/Surveys/fs/en

Variations in risk between nursing settings and nurses

The 2003 NSS found that, among nurses, those working in trusts providing mental health services have the highest levels of reported violence. This is consistent with the NAO's finding that, in 2001/2002, the rate of violent incident reports in mental health and learning disability trusts was two-and-a half times that for all trusts (Healthcare Commission 2004; NAO 2003b: 2). However, perhaps reflecting their primary interest in auditing trusts' overall risk management performance, neither body investigated differences between specific clinical settings within NHS trusts. It has often been suggested that nurses working in acute in-patient mental health care are particularly likely to experience violence. For example, a 2002 survey of such nurses commissioned by the UKCC, specifically concerned with violence, found that three-quarters of respondents reported having been physically assaulted at least once in their careers. But the problem of possible response bias was noted and no comparative data were collected (UKCC 2002).

Interestingly, although the RCN survey cited earlier found that nurses working in learning disabilities and mental health care reported the highest prevalence of harassment and assault in the previous 12 months (49 and 46 per cent), the rates for nurses working in acute adult care and old people's homes were scarcely lower (45 and 44 per cent) (RCN 2002).

Within general hospitals, Accident & Emergency (A&E) departments have often been assumed to bear the brunt of violence (Cembrowicz and Shepherd 1992; Wells and Bowers 2002) but this claim has been questioned (Wells and Bowers 2002; Whittington et al. 1996). A recent survey of front-line staff in one UK general hospital found that nurses in medical departments were more likely to report assaults within the last 12 months than those working in A&E. Threatening behaviour and verbal abuse by patients or visitors were, however, most prevalent in A&E departments (although both these findings should be treated with caution because the overall response rate was only 33 per cent) (Winstanley and Whittington

2004). The same authors have also published a study based on retrospective semi-structured interviews with staff of a general hospital that reported incidents of violence (physical assaults and threats) to the research team over a three-month period. Two-thirds of the incidents reported took place in in-patient wards rather than A&E. In-patient incidents were significantly more likely to involve perpetrators who were female, over 70 years of age and to have had cognitive impairments than those in A&E (Winstanley and Whittington 2002). Suggesting, as they do, that violence may take different forms in different contexts, these two studies underline the value, for both explanation and management of incidents, of distinguishing different types of violence in data collection and analysis, and of collecting contextual information about incidents.

There are few data available on work-related violence against nurses outside large NHS hospitals. And there are also few studies which examine any possible relationships between nurses' social and demographic characteristics and their likelihood of experiencing violence. The UKCC's survey of mental health nurses found that younger, inexperienced nurses were more likely to be physically assaulted, which is in accord with the NSS data on unregistered (including student) nurses and the general conclusions of Wells and Bowers (2002) and Winstanley and Whittington (2004). However, the latter found some indication that, with respect to threatening behaviour, 'if visitors wish to remonstrate, they seem to seek out the most authoritative member of staff available', namely senior nursing grades or doctors (2004: 9). Somewhat surprisingly, the possible significance of nurses' gender or ethnicity in relation to work-related violence is often not considered in research, although the 2003 NSS found that there were no 'meaningful differences' between staff from different ethnic backgrounds in reports of physical or non-physical violence (Healthcare Commission 2004: 50, 52).

To summarise this section, the cumulative weight of quantitative evidence indicates clearly that nursing as an occupation does carry an above average risk of work-related violence. But no precise figure can be placed on the statistical risks of particular kinds of violence facing nurses overall. Furthermore, the available data do not give unequivocal support to the claim quoted in the opening paragraph of this chapter, that nursing is the 'most dangerous job in Britain', or even when compared to ambulance crews and health care assistants, the most dangerous within the NHS. However, as our discussion has indicated, variations in organisational and research definitions, in individual perceptions of what counts as violence, and in propensity to report incidents make any comparisons of rates over time very problematic (except for the generally consistent BCS data). There is little evidence that the actual incidence of physical assaults across the health service has been increasing since the 1990s, which may reflect the impact of preventive measures. Increases in reports of non-physical violence, in particular, may be, in part, artefacts of changes in reporting systems and in propensity to report.

The same problems limit comparison between nursing settings. Those working in mental health care may be more likely to experience physical assault than general nurses as a whole, but overall prevalence rates may conceal considerable variations within organisations. And, as noted above, there are very few qualitative studies of the meaning nurses attribute to aggressive behaviours in different contexts and of their associated responses, or of how nurses undertake risk assessment and manage potentially dangerous interactions (Trenoweth 2003 is a recent exception). The relative risks faced in their work are much debated when nurses from different clinical areas swap 'war stories' (Lee 1995). But, as we have indicated, there is limited evidence with which any arguments might be resolved.

Work-related violence and the 'risk culture'

Whatever are the actual patterns of work-related violence, it is clear that this is an issue that many nurses are currently concerned about. According to recent BCS data, nurses (and other health and welfare associate professionals) are the category of workers most likely to describe themselves as 'very/fairly worried' about assaults (36 per cent) and threats (41 per cent). Asked about the likelihood of being victims of violence in the next 12 months, 28 per cent of this group considered themselves 'very/fairly likely' to be assaulted, and 48 per cent to be threatened. This was, respectively, almost 9 and 21 times more than the actual prevalence rate for assaults and threats reported by this group in the previous 12 months (Upson 2004: 30–36).

How far such worries and expectations arise from directly experienced violence; from changing perceptions of verbal abuse and other acts of non-physical aggression; from raised awareness about reporting violence; or from increased exposure to initiatives aimed at preventing and managing violence, is impossible to determine. But this concern about violence is consonant with the risk culture, the fear and uncertainty characterising contemporary NHS nursing, identified by (Annandale 1996), a culture in which patients are increasingly seen as risk generators. Annandale's key point is that, with the reformulation of patients as consumers with enhanced rights and expectations in successive NHS reforms since the 1980s, new demands for nursing accountability have arisen. These lead in turn to increased self-surveillance, defensive clinical practice and anxiety on the part of nurses. Annandale's focus is primarily on clinical risks, on patient safety and malpractice allegations, but her analysis may also be relevant to work-related violence in several ways. Increasingly demanding consumers with rising expectations figure prominently in many attempts to account for the allegedly growing problem of violence to NHS staff (Hart 2004: 264, NAO 2003a: 2, Oxtoby 2004: 23). That is, the generators of risk are not just from the small group of 'the seriously mad' or 'the very bad', but now potentially from the majority 'normal' public, especially if an inclusive definition of violence is employed. On the one hand, nurses may come to see themselves as more vulnerable to violence as a result of this representation, and associated pressures to be more risk aware. On the other hand, labelling aggressive and offensive behaviour from the public as clearly unacceptable, as warranting negative sanctions, places some responsibility back onto the patient or the employing organisation. The NHS, like all employers, has a legal obligation to ensure, as far as possible, the health and safety of its staff (NAO 2003a). In the final section of this chapter, we present a brief analysis of the policies developed in the NHS for preventing and managing work-related violence, focusing on the national level, showing how these are framed in terms of risk.

Reducing and managing the risk: the NHS – a zero tolerance zone for violence

The first, obvious point to note is the domination of debates about violence in the NHS by the vocabulary of risk assessment and risk management and the constant reference to statistics. As we have indicated, research on work-related violence in healthcare has been primarily concerned with attempts to establish, for logistic reasons, the calculable risk of violence to organisations or occupational groups rather than with individuals or sub-groups within those occupations. However, as we have shown, the validity and reliability of most risk estimates are, at best, open to question. Early initiatives on violence taken by the Labour Government first elected in 1997 required NHS trusts to implement monitoring systems and to achieve National Improvement Targets for reducing incidents of violence and aggression by 20 per cent by 2001, and 30 per cent by 2003 (DoH 1999d). These quantitative targets and monitoring system standards were subsequently incorporated into the ZTZ campaign (DoH 1999c) and the *Improving Working Lives* guidance (DoH 2000b). However, as already indicated, attempts to standardise on a broad definition of violence and, through ZTZ and associated campaigns by nursing and other organisations, to improve incident reporting has led, at least in the short term, to a marked *increase* in recorded violence. By 2003, the NHS in England as a whole had come nowhere near reaching these national targets for incident reduction, although some individual NHS trusts have done so (NAO 2003b). Moreover, the NAO found that, in 2003, implementation of standardised reporting systems was still far from complete across the NHS, and under-reporting was still regarded as a serious problem for NHS risk management (NAO 2003a and b).

Perhaps reflecting the development of risk thinking about violence within the NHS, there has been a recent shift in organisational responsibility for this issue at the central government level. When launched, responsibility for ZTZ lay with the human resources section of the DoH. Work-related violence was conceptualised as primarily a personnel and workforce policy issue: the risks were to individual staff and to the service through the impact of violence on staff well-being, retention and recruitment. In 2003, responsibility for violence passed to the newly established NHS Counter Fraud and Security Management Service (CFSMS). In the words of the CFSMS chief executive, this moved the campaign against violence beyond a 'moral crusade' to being part of a professionalised comprehensive security system for the NHS (Whitfield 2003); 'replicating elements of the approach that CFSMS has taken to tackling fraud and corruption in the NHS' (NHS Executive 2003). Phase V of the ZTZ campaign employed the slogan 'The true costs of harassment' (NHS Executive 2002). Although the poster illustrations are of the emotional costs from abuse to individuals, perhaps the slogan invites consideration of financial damage.

These developments, like the NAO's close scrutiny of violence, are all premised on there being parallels between fraud, waste of public expenditure and violence as risks to the NHS. As such, they appear to resonate with some aspects of the governmentality approach to risk of Rose (1993) and Castel (1991), whose work is discussed in more detail in both Chapter 1 and Chapter 7 of this book. These authors argue that risk thinking in contemporary Britain, characterised by what they term an ideology of advanced liberalism, is bringing about the dissolution of the autonomous acting subject to be replaced by conformity to bureaucratic processes based on abstract calculations. In the case of work-related violence there is potential, in theory at least, for two sets of subjects to be dissolved: nurses, if autonomous practice and the use of professional judgement to manage dangerous situations is displaced by following routinised protocols for risk assessment and management: and the perpetrators of violence.

Our analysis of the discourse on the perpetrators in the ZTZ campaign and related NHS policy guidance suggests that some perpetrators of violence against health care staff are being 'responsibilised' rather than simply dissolved, in line with a general shift in penal policy towards holding offenders fully responsible for their actions (and therefore punishable). As we have argued elsewhere (Elston *et al.* 2002), the emerging dominant stance in policy discourse on violence in the NHS is, ostensibly, a punitive one. 'We don't have to take this – and we didn't' was the message of posters in the 2001 relaunch of ZTZ, accompanied by pictures of newspaper cuttings about successful prosecutions for assaults on NHS staff (NHS Executive 2001a). ZTZ leaflets and web-pages provide extensive guidance on involving the police and using the criminal justice system, with the implication that these should be regarded as normal organisational responses, rather than left mainly to the discretion of individual staff who have been subjected to violence. Decisions about further action, such as criminal prosecution, would then pass to the police and the Crown Prosecution Service. One of the key actions proposed by the CFSMS at its inception was developing 'a Memorandum of Understanding with the Association of Chief Police Officers that sets out what the NHS can expect from the police and what they can expect from the NHS around security, and in particular about dealing with violence and aggression towards staff' (NHS Executive 2003).

Thus, within much ZTZ material, the perpetrators of violence against NHS staff have been represented not, for the most part, as sick and distressed patients unable to help their abusive behaviour and in need of better professional care, but as those against whom the NHS and its staff should be defended. Such deviants may, by their own actions, compromise their entitlement to care, whether or not criminal sanctions are applied. NHS trusts have been required to develop local policies and procedures for withholding treatment from serial perpetrators of violence as a last resort (NHS Executive 2001b) and provision has also been made for such individuals to forfeit their rights to be registered with general practitioners in their immediate locality (Elston *et al.* 2002). The dominant tone is clear: perpetrators who transgress in their interactions with health care professionals risk exclusion from the normal rights of citizenship, in the form of constraints on their access to NHS services. Such exclusion is another theme of the Foucauldian analysis of governmentality and risk in advanced liberalism (Higgs 1998).

Calls to exclude from treatment or criminalise the perpetrators of violence against healthcare staff, appear to stand in sharp contrast to a medicalised model which sees violence as caused by patients' underlying pathology, which may, in turn, warrant absolution of patients from responsibility for their actions. And such calls may strike many readers as contestable in some circumstances, for example, when the perpetrators of violence are elderly, confused women resisting nurses' attempts to bathe or feed them. And it is clear from the detailed analysis of ZTZ measures by the NAO that, within the NHS, prosecutions of assailants and withholding policies are still only pursued in a tiny proportion of recorded instances of violence (NAO 2003b). Thus, for example, it does not appear that mental health nurses who are hit or sworn at by patients in the course of their work are now routinely following general ZTZ guidance by setting in motion the processes that might lead to patient prosecution (Gournay 2002).

In fact, the detailed ZTZ guidance on withholding treatment policies reveals the difficulties of applying an unqualified 'staff as victims to be defended' approach to risk reduction in a public health service. The guidance states that patients who are mentally ill or who might be under the influence of drugs or alcohol should be exempted from such sanctions (NHS Executive 2001b). Determining which violent patients fall into the exempted category is presumably a matter for clinical judgement, appropriately guided by protocols. Those working with acutely disturbed patients in mental health services now have two sets of guidance to resort to: that from ZTZ, with its general, if qualified, emphasis on reducing risk to staff and blaming perpetrators of violence; and that from NICE which places great emphasis on the rights of service users, and sets out protocols for the use of means of restraint, such as seclusion or rapid tranquillisation, which, temporarily at least, violate such rights. The NICE guideline clearly draws on a more medicalised model of violence, focusing on the needs of patients for professional assistance. But, in the aftermath of the 'Rocky' Bennett case, NICE sets out a modified medicalised model that formally inscribes the acutely disturbed mental health service user as a consumer with rights and, when well enough, responsibilities, for example, to agree advance directives as to how s/he would prefer to be treated in the event of becoming highly disturbed (NICE 2005). This is consonant with a suggestion made by Rose (1998, 2000) that, under advanced liberalism, those deviants who pose relatively low risk or offer some prospect of re-insertion into society may be offered quasi-contracts to help in a process of 'ethical reconstruction' under professional surveillance, rather than being totally excluded from health and welfare services (or totally exempted from responsibility).[7]

So, officially promulgated formal policies with respect to work-related violence in the NHS do exhibit many of the characteristics of risk thinking identified by writers on governmentality in advanced liberalism. There is potentially tension between the model of the perpetrator implicit in much of ZTZ and the recognition that many perpetrators may not be wholly responsible for their actions at the time of an incident because of their medical condition. But even policies orientated to medicalised interpretations of violence are incorporating notions of patients as persons with rights and responsibilities to reduce the risk they pose to others.

Conclusion

We have shown how violence in recent years has become recognised as an issue for nurses working in all settings, and that there is clear evidence that nursing is an occupation at relatively high risk of work-related violence. At the same time, our review of the evidence suggests a need to keep a sense of proportion. There is little robust evidence of an increase in actual incidence of physical or non-physical violence in recent years, although this cannot be definitively ruled out. Increased official recognition has been given to so-called 'low-grade' violence such as verbal abuse, although whether effective preventive measures have been implemented is not a question we have attempted to

---

[7] A similar process is occurring in management of patients with substance abuse problems in general practice through the use of quasi-contracts Elston, M. A., Gabe, J., Denney, D., Lee, R., and O'Beirne, M. (2002) 'Violence against doctors: a medical(ised) problem? The case of National Health Service general practitioners', *Sociology of Health and Illness*, 24, 5, 575–598.

address here. One point most researchers on violence agree on is that the evidence-base for effective strategies for preventing and managing violence is weak (Wright *et al.* 2002). We have suggested that the way work-related violence has been framed as a policy issue exemplifies the dominance of the discourse of risk management in contemporary health policy. This is shown by the emphasis on statistics and quantitatively defined targets; the expansion of the category of risk behaviour and of risk generators so that violence comes to be represented as a normal 'risk of the job' but one that 'we don't have to take', as in the ZTZ campaign. The emphasis on responsibilising the perpetrators of violence to NHS staff in recent official policy discourse contrasts, in many respects, with health professionals' traditional medicalised model focusing on the needs of patients for professional clinical assistance (even, or especially, when violent). But the medicalised model itself may be being modified to incorporate patients' rights and responsibilities for their risk generating behaviour.

With respect to the recurrent dilemma between therapeutic management and staff-protection, the official policy pendulum has perhaps swung towards protection of staff in recent years, but the dilemma remains. And analysing official discourses does not tell us how nurses themselves interpret formal policies in their practice, how they act on or resist and transform them in practice and how they themselves deal with the dilemma. These are questions to which we do not yet have good answers.

4 The rise of risk thinking in mental health nursing

Paul Godin

Introduction

Britain has witnessed considerable changes in the organisation of its mental health care services. All but a few Victorian asylums, which had been in inexorable decline since the 1950s, were finally shut down in the late 1980s and 1990s. Since the 1950s, mental health care has been increasingly practised in a wide range of sites; in acute wards, day centres, clinics, nursing homes, supported living schemes, the private homes of mental health service users and amongst the homeless in the street. As Rose (1996) explains, the psychiatric archipelago of the asylum system became far more complex as the asylum islands submerged. Yet professional–client interaction survived and increased on a multitude of new islets. Eventually a policy framework took shape for the delivery of community mental health care, where it was now largely based, out of the *NHS and Community Care Act* (Department of Health (DoH) 1990). This, along with all other contemporary mental health care policy and practice, has come to be dominated by a concern about the rational assessment and management of risk; what Rose (1998) terms 'risk thinking'.

In this chapter, I argue that this recent rise of 'risk thinking' represents a profound transformation of mental health care. Many mental health care nurses and other mental health care professionals might regard the new emphasis on risk assessment and risk management as a relatively insignificant appendage to their work. However, I contend that it is at the heart of what orders contemporary mental health care practice and makes it distinctly different from what preceded it. This contention is based upon Castel's thesis that the mental health system has, over two centuries, developed and refined its methods of dealing with the threat of madness, finally surpassing the 'clinic of the subject' (focused on danger and disease within individual patients) to spawn the 'epidemiological clinic' (focused on risk factors within populations). This transformation is far from complete, and there are enough vestiges of the 'clinic of the subject' to give us the false impression that the rise in risk thinking within mental care is only a mundane and unimportant feature of contemporary mental health care practice. However, I argue that this rational, calculative control of madness is having a profound and irreversible effect on service users and mental health care workers.

It is often assumed that the risk thinking was born of a growing public concern about the danger of mental patients at large within society, fuelled by public awareness of the fact that the old asylums were now finally being closed down. Sharkey (2000), in a text book on Community Care, contends that concern about the Sharon Campbell case (in which a mental patient knifed to death her former social worker) led to the introduction of the risk management regime of care programme approach (CPA) in community mental health care. Though I do not dispute that this was a relevant factor, the development of the new regime of community mental health care of the 1990s needs to be understood within a broader historical and social context, which Castel's thesis provides. Therefore, following Castel's thesis, I first outline how modern psychiatry moved from thought about danger to risk thinking and how the latter orders the present regime of mental health care, the epidemiological clinic. I then consider what effect the epidemiological clinic is having on mental health service users and professionals before lastly speculating on what its development might mean for the future.

Dangerousness to risk

Castel did much to advance Foucault's work. Whereas Foucault (1971) had written a pre-history of modern psychiatry (modern meaning the last 200 years), Castel tells the story of modern psychiatry. In so doing, he advances Foucault's concept of governmentality (Foucault 1991), emphasising how mental health care of the modern era has been intrinsically bound up with the problematics, techniques and practices of liberal rule. Psychiatry has reflected the values and methods of rule that distinguished in turn, laissez-faire liberalism, welfare liberalism and advanced liberalism. In this development Castel discerns a rationalising trend within mental health care, in its *preventive* strategies, towards the control of the threat of madness, from the confinement of those declared insane, and thus *dangerous*, to the efficient control of *risk* factors within the population.

Castel's history of modern psychiatry is based largely on the case of France and the United States of America (USA). Therefore, in examining Castel's account of how the preventive strategies of mental health care developed, I endeavour to paint British mental health care into his picture. I also draw on the work of other historians of mental health care to examine the historical claims made by Castel's thesis. I consider, in turn, how the preventive strategy of mental health care shifted from confinement to elimination and then to generalised intervention, and now to highly rational methods of risk profiling patients and their assignment to care/risk management programmes.

Confinement

For both Foucault and Castel, it was the rise of moral treatment that distinguished the beginning of psychiatry in the modern era. In seeking to moralise, civilise and restore the productive capacity of patients, moral treatment reflected the values of emergent liberal society of the late eighteenth century. The nineteenth-century asylum system, which in Britain was modelled on the York Retreat (a pioneering centre of excellence for moral treatment), became the basis for psychiatry's development as a medical discipline, where it refined its nosologies and taxonomies. Though Castel calls this the 'golden age of psychiatry' (1988) it operated a very crude method of dealing with the threat of madness. Danger was assumed to be an immanent yet intrinsic quality of insanity. Within what Castel (1991) calls 'classical psychiatry', it was commonly assumed that both insanity and danger were embodied in the patient. Once insanity had been identified, it followed that confinement was necessary to prevent the eruption of the danger associated with it. As psychiatry only confined a minority of the people that it could potentially identify as insane, whose propensity to violence was only ever assumed rather than known, this was a very crude and highly inefficient method of dealing with the threat of madness. This failure was popularly known and mocked in the old adage 'there's more out than in'.

Castel identifies Morel as a nineteenth-century psychiatrist with a vision for a more effective strategy of prevention. Morel had suggested that public authorities undertake special surveillance amongst the 'subproletariat', to identify and act on the conditions liable to produce their high risk of mental illness, namely malnutrition, alcoholism, housing conditions, sexual promiscuity, and so on. Though his idea was not realised, as there was not then the means at the disposal of psychiatry to achieve this ambition, Morel was 'already arguing in terms of *objective risks:* that is to say, statistical correlation between series of phenomena' (Castel 1991: 284). However, objective risk thinking came to be realised in a somewhat different form in the first half of the twentieth century.

Elimination

From the late nineteenth century the psychiatric ideology of degeneracy, otherwise referred to as 'psychiatric Darwinism', increasingly gained popularity. An accumulating population of incurable in-mates came to be seen as the result of a wider social malaise. Mental illness was increasingly identified as an inherited disease that gave rise to degenerative behaviour, which worsened the patient's condition and that of any offspring they might bare, to whom, it was believed, they were highly likely to transmit the disease. This psychiatric ideology, that reflected the values of the time, amongst those with wealth, power and influence, gave rise to eugenic policies in the twentieth century. Eugenics also involved reasoning in terms of risk rather than danger. Through its technologies of sterilisation and euthanasia, eugenics promised to prevent the risk of mental illness being transmitted from one generation to the next. Unlike confinement, the elimination technologies of eugenics suppressed future risk rather than just present danger.

The Nazi regime, in which eugenics was realised, had a considerable effect upon European psychiatric populations. Bennett (1991: 631) estimates there to have been between 70,000 and 120,000 mental patients killed in Nazis Germany and between 200,000 and 350,000 compulsorily sterilised. The technologies of extermination practiced in the Nazis death camps were first developed in the German asylums. Goodwin (1997) points to a reduction in the French psychiatric in-patient population from 115,000 before the war to 65,000 afterwards; much of which, Barham (1992) points out, occurred in Vichy France, where in-mates were deliberately starved.

Even prior to the rise of Nazi Germany in the early twentieth century, eugenic policy and practice was widespread. Kevles (1985) notes that by 1930 twenty-four states within the USA had laws on their statute books allowing for the forced sterilisation of mental patients. Though British psychiatry was never subject to eugenic policies, I suggest that the psychiatric ideology of degeneracy led to elimination through starvation. Minimal spending on asylums led to patients being held in poor conditions of near starvation, which became particularly severe during the First World War as the asylum budgets were halved (Raftery 1996: 26). There was a dramatic increase in the asylum death rate during the war till in 1918 a third of the asylum population of England and Wales died in the space of one twelve month period (17,293 in excess of the average ratio for asylums for the preceding decade (Lomax 1921: 32–3)). Against the long-term trend of an ever increasing asylum population, the asylum population briefly declined. The Board of Control (a body that then monitored standards within the asylums of England and Wales) reported that in 1918 influenza (then becoming a Europe wide pandemic) and tuberculosis had accounted for 1217 and 1021 of these asylum deaths respectively (Lomax 1921: 61). Lomax, an asylum doctor, thus comments 'I wonder if it had ever occurred to these learned gentlemen [members of the board of control] to connect this excessive mortality with the facts of deficient clothing and defective feeding' (Lomax 1921: 61). His personal account of working as an asylum doctor during the First World War, testifies to the practice of deprivation and starvation of asylum in-mates and their resulting exceptionally high death rate. The ideology of degeneracy led to contemptuous and negligent treatment of the English asylum in-mate population towards their elimination around the period of the First World War.

Elimination, inspired by ideologies of degeneracy, social Darwinism and eugenics, was finally halted as their scientific and moral basis were questioned in the wake of the defeat of Nazi Germany. Industrialised nations, such as Britain, set about establishing state welfare and new social rights for its citizens on a large scale, which decisively shifted liberal societies into an era of 'welfare liberalism'. As health and welfare became more freely available and more clearly the responsibility of the state, psychiatry was able to widen its mandate beyond the treatment of the mentally ill. Accordingly, it was from here onward that the term 'mental health care' gained more general parlance. Similarly, social work no longer attended exclusively to the needs of the poor. The preventive strategy of psychiatry thus moved to one of generalised intervention.

Generalised intervention

Castel (1991) notes how the model of 'Preventive Psychiatry', advanced by Gerald Caplan (1964), provided a blueprint for the USA's radical shift towards community mental health care, to realise Morel's aspirations of 100 years before, to act directly on the conditions within society that were liable to produce the risk of mental illness. Britain's move towards community care and generalised intervention of mental health care was slower than that in the USA and informed rather by 'social psychiatry' than preventive psychiatry. However, Britain did later, in the 1980s, begin to emulate the American Community Mental Health Centre Model, predicated on Caplan's preventive psychiatry. Though there are differences between post-Second World War mental health care in Britain and the USA, both distinctly involved a widening of mental health care interventions to the entire population.

Castel describes how Caplan's model helped broaden the role of psychiatry in a fundamental shift of its preventive strategy. Caplan distinguished three levels at which psychiatry could prevent mental illness, supporting an expanding role for psychiatry. In reverse order, tertiary prevention was aimed at minimising the disabling effects of mental illness; secondary prevention aimed to avert the development of mental illness through early intervention in the lives of people undergoing personal crises and, most radically, primary prevention was to deal with the conditions that gave rise to mental illness. Through changing the practices of government agencies and laws a whole programme of political intervention was to control factors that both give rise to mental illness and promote good mental health. Mental health care was no longer just something that the state delegated to mental health care professionals but was now also part of state policy and its administration.

Caplan's account of primary prevention articulates the essence of this new role of mental health care, enmeshed in the state's administrative system that aims to control risk factors within a generalised space. Castel explains this move towards 'the new space of risk':

> the notion of risk is made autonomous from danger. A risk does not arise from the presence of particular precise danger embodied in a concrete individual or group. It is the effect of a combination of abstract factors which render more or less probable the occurrence of undesirable modes of behaviour. (1991: 287)

He argues that it has given rise to a *'new mode of surveillance:* that of systematic prediction' (Castel 1991: 288). It primarily targets factors rather than individuals, though through such scientific prediction certain individuals may be identified with a certain number of risk factors that warrant investigation and possible treatment.

This new mode of surveillance has been made possible by a steady increase in health checks and records that, Castel points out, make patients' dossiers the focus of examination, rather than the physically present subject. Presence has been replaced by memory in a shift from the clinical gaze to the objective accumulation of facts. The disciplinary relationship in the clinic of the subject between the carer and cared for, in face-to-face relationships, has been replaced by a new epidemiological clinic that attends to factors within the population. This new strategy has dissolved the notion of the subject.

Does Castel, perhaps, misrepresent or exaggerate the changes that have taken place in post-Second World War mental health care? There has surely been a growth rather than decline in the practices of the clinic of the subject. Many more mental health care professionals attend to many more people with mental health needs in face-to-face relationships than was the case before the demise of the asylum. Though record keeping might now consume more of professionals' time and might form the basis of assessment more than physically present patients, intensely individualised forms of clinical practice, such as Assertive Community Treatment and Home Treatment have developed.

Castel is, perhaps, guilty of overlooking a point that Dean (1997) makes, namely that risk groups, such as the 'seriously mentally ill', are now subject to highly intensive face-to-face case management. However, Castel outlines a profound transformation in mental health care practice that is particularly apparent in the mental health policy and practices of the era of neo-liberalism, in which mental health service users are profiled by risk assessment and then assigned to a social trajectory that mental health care professionals help/persuade/coerce their clients to follow.

Risk profiling and care programmes

Having identified the shift towards the epidemiological clinic, Castel expressed grave concerns about its future. He explains how the community mental health centre model, which enabled mental health care practice to expand and reach a maximum number of people, is now changing in the new era of neo-liberalism, towards the projection, rather than just the imposition, of social order. The scientific prediction that emerged with psychiatry's more generalised intervention is developing further towards the 'absolute reign of calculative reason', in which individual's potential to function within the condition of neo-liberalism is profiled. From this profile they are invited to follow a set career, laid out in advance for them, that will ensure maximum efficiency, for as Castel asserts, this new order is obsessed with efficiency rather than discipline.

It is here that Castel is most prescient; for he aptly describes the new system of community mental health care that is taking shape in Britain. Since the introduction of Care Programme Approach (CPA), an administrative system has arisen to ensure that all mental health care service users are risk profiled, through the use of a growing battery of risk assessment measures, and then assigned a social destiny (a care programme) to secure their safe conduct, through deploying the most efficient use of mental health care services resources. Stable patients, requiring a basic level of care, are placed on 'standard CPA'. If their stability continues, pressure mounts for them to be discharged to primary care. Patients whose risk profile indicates that they need complex care from more than one mental health practitioner are assigned to 'enhanced CPA'. Community supervision and restriction orders are used to monitor the conduct of patients in the community whose risk profiles pose particularly high risk.

The psychiatric in-patient population is also graded by patients' risk profiles. Psychiatric Intensive Care Units (PICUs) have been developed within acute in-patient care areas to accommodate patients that come to pose a high risk within the acute sector. The special hospitals, now known as high security hospitals, have been supplemented with regional secure units, providing medium and low security care. In all parts of the system, patients are risk profiled and assigned a destiny (care plan), designed to minimise their level of risk, which is monitored and adjusted as they are re-profiled.

In the era of generalised intervention, psychiatry had freely broadened its mandate to provide what Caplan described as 'comprehensive mental health care'. This fairly indiscriminate application of mental health care service ended with the shift towards the risk profiling of service users, which provided a logical imperative to support the prioritisation of services. However, this move from generalised to targeted interventions was based less on any concept of need, that obliged professionals to offer extensive provision, than on the level of threat posed by the patient. Risk assessment is tacitly and conveniently assumed to encompass what a client needs, whilst medical diagnosis and treatment have become just one part of the greater process of risk assessment and risk management.

Mental health care service users in the epidemiological clinic

Are service users better or worse off within the present regime of the epidemiological clinic than they were before? Surely being a service user today is preferable to the confinement and elimination of the past. For all the social exclusion and marginalisation that commonly accompanies service users' experience of community care, it is surely preferable to being locked up, starved, sterilised or exterminated. However, without getting overly nostalgic about the mental health care of the welfare liberal era that inaugurated generalised intervention and community care, the neo-liberal development of the epidemiological clinic presents some worrying trends for service users.

First, Castel (1991) contends that as the clinic of the subject is lost so too is care for individuals, for in the epidemiological clinic caring gives way to the expertise of managing risk. Mental health care professionals' growing preoccupation with risk thinking persuades them to regard service users primarily as objects carrying risk factors. Risk assessment tools shape the thinking of nurses and other mental health care workers into prioritising concern about patients' risk of violence and self-harm. Caring about the service users' general well-being becomes a secondary concern for professionals, though remains of primary importance for service users. Caring remains a core value amongst nurses, seen as that which defines their professional purpose. Many nurses will probably disagree angrily with this contention. However, would any mental health care nurses disagree that their caring function is at times, perhaps frequently, compromised by the imperatives of risk thinking?

Second, mental health workers now work within an administrative system that demands to be endlessly fed with data, about care planning, risk assessment, risk management, and outcomes. Though the data are, in part, supposed to measure good patient care, the collection of data (rather than the patients) becomes an end in itself as Trusts strive to maintain and improve their star ratings. Concern about caring for the individual is lost further as much of the data measures population factors. For example, suicide rates, rather than individual cases of suicide, are the object of concern for the mental health care system, as reduction of suicide rates feature as targets for services to achieve. Service users might not be entirely wrong in thinking that professionals, within such a system, are inclined to care about them as a statistic rather than as an individual.

Third, to some extent, as Castel (1991) claims, the epidemiological clinic has now dissolved the notion of the subject and the face-to-face, professional/patient relationship. In the era of generalised intervention people claiming to be suffering mental ill health, rather than a 'serious' mental illness, or to be in personal crisis, were far more likely to be able to secure the attention of a mental health care worker. The prioritisation of those with high risk profiles now ensures that those so qualified are most likely to attract the individual care of a mental health care professional. Low risk people are increasingly managed at a distance from the formal mental health care services, within primary care, through NHS Direct, on phone help lines, on radio phone-in programmes, in TV talk shows and through their own self-management. However, perhaps low risk people, with 'minor' mental illness or in personal crisis, are better off without care/therapy/individual discipline/paternalistic control from mental health care professionals.

Lastly, though high risk mental patients often receive highly individualised and intensive forms of care, such as assertive community treatment and home treatment, it is primarily directed towards ensuring that the patient follows the care pathway set for them, to systematically reduce their level of risk. Progression along the pathway can be slow and frustrating, for not only the patient but also for their professional carer. Consider, for example how, in an interview study of community mental health nurses (CMHNs) perceptions' of risk, a respondent describes the care of his client:

> We've developed this emphasis upon not wanting to make mistakes. And the client has suffered as a result. Before, they had to deal with the

label of being mentally ill, now they're seen as a risk. And professionals are less likely to take therapeutic risks with clients ... their [patients'] history prevents them being considered for things in the future. The doors shut for them. They won't be given the chance again. This bloke went into an independent living scheme and relapsed and went into hospital, and was not allowed back to his home, and went into supported care, which he didn't like. And only now, four years later, is he being considered for independent living again. It may fail but he should be given a chance. (Godin 2004: 356)

Notice how the CMHN begins by pointing out that once patients were simply labelled (and followed what Goffman (1970) termed a 'moral career', given by their 'spoilt identity'). Now, the CMHN informs us, patients are seen as a risk, and accordingly have to also follow a career of being risk managed. This rational social trajectory management of clients in the community has, perhaps, created an 'iron cage', which prevents patients from adventurously taking risks and benefiting from the advantages that might ensue. As the CMHN in the above quotation laments, mental health care workers of today will not take the risk of therapeutic risk taking. The CMHN also clearly describes how the risk assessment of the patient renders him a prisoner of his past, having to serve time to improve his profile to then achieve a more autonomous and desirable living situation.

Mental health professionals in the epidemiological clinic

Castel (1991) asserts that in the development of the epidemiological clinic psychiatrists have lost their professional autonomy. In the past, particularly in their 'golden age', psychiatrists had almost complete command over the control of madness. However, as we have seen, in the era of welfare liberalism, the mandate of psychiatry widened and increasingly became a function of state policy and administration. In the neo-liberal era psychiatrists became increasingly subordinate to state administration that augmented its power over mental health care professionals through the collection and monitoring of data about their clients and practice, such that mental health care workers are now functionaries of the mental health care administrative system. Quite simply, knowledge about mental health and the management of it is now less in the hands of psychiatrists and increasingly at the level of administration above them.

If Castel is correct in his thesis, then the high level of professional autonomy that psychiatrists once enjoyed, and that other mental health care occupational groups strove for, has been lost forever. Professional power can give rise to patriarchal domination of their clients and the realisation of professional interests at the expense of patients. Therefore, the loss of professional power is, perhaps, not a bad thing. However, as Castel points out, mental health care professionals have, on occasions, used their autonomy to redirect very positively their mandate to control madness. Castel cites Italian democratic psychiatry's achievements in bringing about community mental health care as an example.

Though professional power is not to be restored, we might ask is the power of the rational system of risk thinking that has replaced it any better? As I have already indicated, it has many negative features for service users. Apart from its limitation on all that is both bad and good about professional power, it also has negative effects on service providers similar to those affecting service users. Mental health care workers are also frustrated with a system that requires them to regard their clients as objects of risk, crowding out care for the well-being of individuals. They become frustrated with feeding data into the system and its disapproval of therapeutic risk taking.

Conclusion

In conclusion, I ask, and attempt to answer, the question of where do we go from here? Castel's thesis clearly indicates that the shift in modern psychiatry from dangerousness to risk, from the clinic of the subject to the epidemiological clinic, heads towards ever more rational methods in the control of the threat of madness. It is unlikely that mental health care could return to its methods of previous eras. Furthermore, many of the practices in these eras, such as confinement and elimination, could hardly be considered desirable. Then, are we stuck in a highly rational system of mental health care in which caring has been transposed into the rational risk assessment and risk management? I suggest that mental health care workers, frustrated by the risk thinking of the neo-liberal epidemiological clinic, have grounds for optimism about the future.

First, it is not a bureaucracy, of the ideal type described by Weber (1948), that mental health workers operate within. The welfare liberalist command and control structure of the National Health Service (NHS) has, in the age of neo-liberalism, given way to a structure that relies less on authority and discipline and more on self-government. The state is far more distant in government as both service users and service providers are encouraged to be active in their own self-government. Therefore, mental health care workers are allowed discretion in how, amongst other things, they assess and manage risk. They could use this discretion to broaden the concept of risk to incorporate what might be seen as patients' needs and wants, to redefine them as risks that would, as such, merit attention. For example, mental health care workers might include in their measurement of risks: the risk of poverty, the risk of being denied choice in service provision and the risk of being denied opportunities for therapeutic risk taking. In doing so, mental health care workers might be able to change risk thinking into a discourse that includes the things that services users are concerned about. Through such redirection of risk thinking nurses might be able to reassert their professional mission of caring.

Second, though risk thinking has a certain compatibility with the values and methods of neo-liberal rule, as we have seen, liberalism is constantly changing. Laissez-faire liberalism lost favour to welfare liberalism, which, in turn, lost favour to neo-liberalism. A widespread expression of discontent with all that is undesirable with risk thinking and neo-liberalist rule in general, could lead to a transformation into an alternative regime that better suited the values and wishes of service users and providers.

5 Different understandings of risk within a forensic mental health care unit: a cultural approach

Paul Godin, Jacqueline Davies,
Bob Heyman and
Monica Shaw

Introduction

This chapter is inspired by our experiences of undertaking a three-year qualitative study of the staff and patients within a medium secure forensic mental health unit, hereafter referred to as 'the Unit' (Heyman *et al.* 2004). In the course of our study, we became increasingly aware that the risk mentally disordered offenders (MDOs) pose to society, which the Unit existed to contain and rehabilitate, and the associated risks that the staff and patients encountered in this risk management of MDOs, were understood and dealt with very differently by people according to their relative position within the organisation. In brief, staff within the Unit's hierarchy had different ideas about what risks MDOs posed and how these risks should be managed. Consequently, some staff felt at risk of exposure to potential violence from the patients, whilst others battled against the risk being identified as failing to do their job properly. Meanwhile, patients felt they were at risk of being harmed by the organisation. We asked ourselves, was it possible that, as Douglas (1992) contends, such variations in risk thinking were the product of social processes of integration (group) and regulation (grid)? In this chapter, we attempt to answer this question as we apply Douglas's grid/group analysis (outlined in the introductory chapter) in our account of how a plurality of risk thinking and associated actions were socially shaped within the medium secure unit we studied. Before doing so, we first consider how Douglas's ideas can inform an understanding of the social context in which medium secure units have come to operate as a major means of control of MDOs.

The city under threat

In the introductory chapter, it is explained how Douglas applied her grid/group model to understand how social integration and regulation shaped a diversity of risk thinking and associated behaviour in the City that was confronted with the grave threat of AIDS in the 1980s. In many respects the city threatened by AIDS is very similar to the city that is now threatened by deinstitutionalised madness. Both threats engendered moral panic within the central community that feared its destruction at the hands of an external force. In the case of the city threatened by deinstitutionalised madness, an image was promoted of menacing mental patients, at large within the city: out of control, a danger to themselves and others. The high profile and frequently retold news story of Christopher Clunis (a black, single and unemployed man) stabbing Jonathan Zito to death (a white, recently married musician) at Finsbury Park underground station in 1992, just prior to Christmas, epitomised the central community's fears about the external threat of madness that had been relocated in its midst. Somebody, with an abundance of attributes demonstrating him to be an outsider, killed a person with all the worthy membership attributes of the central community.

In this climate of fear, government mental health policy aimed to reassure the central community by ensuring that there is effective risk management and control of mental patients. New powers of arrest were afforded to mental health professionals through the introduction of supervised discharge (Department of Health (DoH) 1995). Also, forthcoming legislation is likely to introduce compulsory treatment orders that can be as readily applied to patients in the community as they are to patients in hospital (DoH 2004b). Furthermore, this proposed change in law would also allow for the preventive detention of people defined as having a 'dangerous and severe personality disorder' (DSPD).

Ahead of these legislative changes, new high secure specialist centres have already been opened to accommodate people identified as having DSPD, expanding still further the number of secure psychiatric in-patient places. The last two decades has seen a slow but steady increase in the number of secure places in what are called both 'regional' and 'medium' secure units. These units were originally intended to replace the outdated isolated high security special hospitals (Broadmoor, Rampton and Ashworth), formerly known as criminal lunatic asylums (Home Office and DHSS 1975). However, there has been only a modest decline in the number of MDOs within the special hospitals, which has remained slightly above 1000 since the early 1990s, whilst the number of MDOs in the newly built secure units has increased unremittingly, doubling from 1050 in 1993 to 2015 in 2003 (Ly and Howard 2004). In short, secure provision, in the form of new secure units, has expanded to serve as a major means to control particularly threatening mental patients (namely MDOs) for the protection of the central community.

The unit

This chapter explores the social processes that influence how staff and patients in one of these secure units understand and perform the organisation's function of managing the risk of MDOs. Data were collected through observations, field visits, qualitative interviews, patient-centred case studies and staff seminars. For most of the research period, up to 90 patients were accommodated in 7 wards with an average of 12 beds per ward. The Unit was located on three sites, with varying levels of security. Approximately 150 nurses managed the day-to-day care for patients whilst six consultant-led multi-disciplinary teams (MDTs), each with a hierarchy of doctors, a psychologist, occupational therapist (OT) and social worker, providing assessment and treatment. Over the three years of data collection there has been a rapid turnover of staff. For example, there have been three general managers.

Our extensive interviews generated a large amount of talk about people's thoughts and actions. However, as Douglas (1992: 103) points out, observation of action is vital for any cultural analysis, for in action people demonstrate commitment to the beliefs and values they espouse. Thus, observation of action enabled us to understand exactly which of the beliefs that participants expressed in talk really did direct their actions. Over the course of our three-year study, we accumulated a considerable amount of data about the actions of staff and patients that were observed incidentally whilst visiting the Unit. Our field notes included data about the case conferences we attended and the staff meetings and seminars in which we reported our findings. Also, a multi-disciplinary team workshop provided a particularly rich source of observational data.

Grid/group analysis

We now explain and apply Douglas's grid/group model to demonstrate how staff and patients within the Unit variously understood and dealt with risk. Douglas's grid/group model delineates four ideal type extreme positions given by the two indexes, which chart a two-dimensional map (as illustrated below in Figure 5.1).

As explained in the introductory chapter, Douglas (1992) argues that the cultural position of a society, organisation or individual within this map will give rise to a particular perception, understanding and approach to risk. We now outline how staff and patients of the Unit are positioned within this map.

The grid/group map of the Unit

Grid gap: Before describing our research findings in the context of the four ideal type positions of a grid/group map (as illustrated in Figure 5.1) it is worth noting a striking feature about how patients and staff of the Unit were positioned in

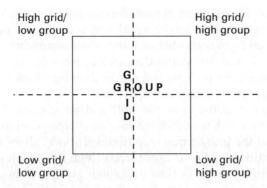

Figure 5.1   Basic grid/Group map

terms of the vertical grid index. In the high grid position patients could hardly be any more constrained and disadvantaged. Our patient-centred case study data revealed that they had often suffered abuse, privation and rule-governed institutional care in their childhood, and are now experiencing highly rule-governed, constrained and unenviable adult lives. By contrast, many of those who cared for them, and to a large extent determined their fate, displayed a far more auspicious social position, through their fine clothes, smart cars, educated accents and professional careers. However, there was also a conspicuous gap between the grid position of nursing staff and the doctors, who were respectively at either end of a steep hierarchy of occupational groups within the Unit.

Nurses largely carried out the work of maintaining security within the Unit. This function, which largely defined their role, rendered them subject to rule-governed procedures that were used to regulate the lives of the patients also controlled them. Though all staff claimed to share an ideal of MDT working, some other professionals indicated that they did not regard nurses as full members of the MDT of professional therapists; in their view, nurses were incapable of providing therapy. In an individual interview, an OT opined that nurses hindered therapy as they conducted their custodial role in an 'iatrogenic' manner. In the MDT workshop (attended by one administrator, three OTs and sixteen nurses), nurses vented frustration about being regarded as an atherapeutic, or even anti-therapeutic, and servile workforce. It might also be noted that this grid gap coincided with the ethnic stratification of the Unit. Black and Asian ethnic minorities were far more prevalent amongst the patients and nurses than they were amongst the OTs, social workers and doctors.

We now consider how the staff and patients of the Unit were located within each of the four ideal type positions at the corners of the grid/group map outlined above, characterising each position as follows: bureaucrats (high grid/high group), the dissenting enclaves (low grid/high group), individualists (low grid/low group) and isolates (high grid/low group), as a diagrammatic summary (see Figure 5.2).

Bureaucrats (blame and risk blindness): The Unit, like most health care organisations in England, is hierarchically

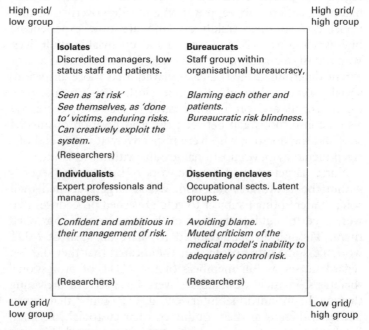

High grid/ low group

High grid/ high group

Isolates
Discredited managers, low status staff and patients.

*Seen as 'at risk'
See themselves, as 'done to' victims, enduring risks. Can creatively exploit the system.*

(Researchers)

Bureaucrats
Staff group within organisational bureaucracy,

*Blaming each other and patients.
Bureaucratic risk blindness.*

Individualists
Expert professionals and managers.

Confident and ambitious in their management of risk.

(Researchers)

Dissenting enclaves
Occupational sects. Latent groups.

*Avoiding blame.
Muted criticism of the medical model's inability to adequately control risk.*

(Researchers)

Low grid/ low group

Low grid/ high group

Figure 5.2   Grid/group map of the unit

structured within and between occupational groups. Though all staff were subject to the rules of the organisation, those at the less powerful end of its hierarchy were particularly rule governed, with little opportunity to exercise autonomy in a high grid position. Yet the rules of an organisation serve to integrate those that operate them, such that they were also in a high group position. Thus the staff that operated the bureaucracy of the Unit can be appropriately located in a high grid/ high group in the top right position of our grid/ group map.

Though the rules might have made for a degree of social solidarity within this staff group there was little trust between the occupational groups. Given the substantial grid gap between lower and higher level staff this was hardly surprising. Their lack of social cohesion was very apparent in their response to their failures. Patients frequently failed to succeed in therapy and rehabilitation. Security was breached on occasions and patients escaped. Patients also self-harmed, destroyed property and assaulted staff. In explanations of these events, the staff variously distributed blame onto each other and the patients. It was believed, particularly at the lower end of the hierarchy, that blame generally got distributed downwards. A nurse consultant who also recognised this trend explained:

> 'cause nursing here is traditional, when there's been a cock-up or a mistake they're [nurses] the ones that bend down and touch their toes and all other professionals come along and give them a good kick. (Nurse Consultant Nicholas, individual general interview)

Official investigations into 'cock-ups', more formally referred to as 'serious untoward incidents' (SUIs), often resulted in staff, particularly nurses, being suspended. This threat of being identified as failing to ensure safety and security within the Unit was a danger that staff of the Unit continually had to live with. Though this omnipresent risk was not discussed very much in staff interviews, in the MDT workshop an OT commented that, following SUIs, staff groups commonly blamed each other. He stated that this led to each discipline retreating within the boundaries of its respective professional group, which prevented inter-disciplinary collaboration and MDT practice.

> people are blamed and you know, the nurses start being particularly blamed and things. And then it makes their experience of the thing … it's extremely difficult for them to sort of maintain their, um, sort of prominence, you know, role and significance in the MDT. [Talking together] You know there is a fear of actually engaging in the MDT process because that is actually a potential for further blame. (OT Toby, MDT workshop)

Many of the staff interviewed explained that the aim of the Unit was very difficult to achieve, given the nature of the client group. Some nurses expressed the view that the Unit could not properly function because it cared for too many subversive clients, who were bad rather than mad. Such patients, it was claimed, turned the organisation from a hospital into a prison (from a respectable to degenerative institution), subverting the integrity, moral status and main task of the Unit and its ability to function. As one nurse manager put it:

> you get what we call 'prison behaviour', you know, their illness is not clear-cut and then they get into what we call 'jailing behaviour' which is about manipulation; it's about subversion so that's about splitting the staff and they [patients] start bringing drugs and alcohol into the Unit. (Nurse Manager Norman, individual general interview)

Though staff commonly expressed the view that the organisational framework did not adequately control the risk of the clients they cared for, this was largely regarded as a failing in how procedures were operated, rather than as an inherent deficiency of the organisation's routinised bureaucratic approach. Nurses on the wards protested that breaches of security were largely the result of their not having enough staff to implement procedures properly and safely. Doctors and senior nurses commonly proposed that it was rather the stupidity and incompetence of ward nurses that were to blame.

Yet, as Rayner (1986) demonstrates, through example of health professionals dealing with radiological hazards, even if routinised bureaucratic risk procedures are made to work properly, they will not eliminate all risk, for they encourage a selective process of emphasising some risks whilst ignoring others. Those operating the bureaucratic procedures become blind to risks that the organisational framework does not recognise.

Such bureaucratic risk blindness became apparent in a seminar in which we presented some of our findings to a group of staff. One finding presented was that, in interviews, staff had described how patients 'sabotaged' their progress. Interview participants suggested that, though patients commonly expressed a strong desire to be discharged, they were also fearful of freedom and often unconsciously 'messed up' so as to upset their progress. When discussing this finding, one nurse described this phenomenon as 'gate fever'. Presentation of this finding in the seminar evoked staff discussion about a patient who had recently attempted to escape from a first floor rehabilitation ward, just days before he was to be discharged from the Unit. In the escape attempt the patient had fallen and sustained serious physical injuries. An internal inquiry was underway to investigate this SUI and a number of nursing staff had been suspended. In the seminar group, a doctor (Helena) proposed that such knowledge about patients' inclination to sabotage their progress should have made the nurses especially vigilant in their observation of the patient. A nurse responded by protesting that they were not at fault as the patient had been assessed as being of low risk and was therefore on low-level observation. The organisational framework seemingly processed patients in a rational fashion from high risk and high security to low risk and low security. Patients were understood to be at a particular point on this continuum and could not be understood as ambiguously and simultaneously at various points along it. This rational routinised bureaucracy did not have a mechanism for conceptualising and dealing with patients' irrational behaviour, such as 'gate fever'. Ironically, though staff commonly recognised its existence they were blind to it in their operation of the bureaucratic framework; all, that is, except for the doctor who, as an individual removed from the routine procedures of security, could be critical of the nurses seeing, but not seeing this risk.

Dissenting enclaves (muted voices): As OT Toby said (above), when blame was to be distributed, professionals commonly retreat within the boundaries of their own disciplinary grouping. In these enclaves professionals sought to avoid the heavy burden of blame that needed to be deposited some-where.

A degree of dissent could be heard from within the various professional enclaves against the medical model, which was believed by many to dominate in the Unit to the detriment of good service provision. With a hint of defensiveness (towards blaming doctors), the nurses who attended the MDT work-shop protested this claim throughout the day. For example, they claimed that patients had a multitude of problems apart from their mental illness, such as drug and alcohol misuse, which led them into offending behaviour which was only partially addressed by a narrow medical model, which they accused psychiatrists of taking. This, the nurses claimed, resulted in patients being declared mentally well and dis-charged only to re-offend shortly afterwards. This complaint that the medical model was limited in its ability to attend to the risks patients posed was also voiced in many individual interviews with OTs and social workers as well as nurses. However, in the ward rounds and MDT clinical meetings we observed, nobody protested that psychiatrists were taking a too limited medical approach. There was little disagreement about how patients' needs were defined or how they should be best met, other than between the doctors and psycholo-gists. Though a voice resonated from below, about how the domination of the medical model led to the Unit's inability to be more successful in its management of the full range of risks posed by MDOs, this view was not articulated within MDT meetings.

Douglas (1986) points out that enclaves are frequently undeveloped, rather than substantially real, as 'latent groups' that fail to coalesce, not possessing the powerful array of influ-ences, such as coercion, that complex hierarchies employ to induce individual commitment. In particular, we suggest that the steep gradient of the hierarchy within this organisation helped mute these dissenting voices. Unqualified nurses were not even allowed a presence in MDT meetings. Though a journal club existed for inter-professional development, doc-tors had only recently allowed nurses to attend. The hierarchy appeared to inhibit the development of any occupational sect or other grouping from forming a dissenting enclave.

Though some of the patients interviewed voiced dissenting views and opposition to the organisation, they could better be regarded as isolates than a dissenting enclave. Outside the staff hierarchy, in their high grid position, their views could be easily pathologised and otherwise discredited by the staff. The patients of the Unit had insufficient capital of any form, least of all symbolic capital, to exert power and influence within the system, except to cause havoc. They were unable to organise themselves into an effective group, other than as disruptive gangs, described by the staff as indicative of these patients' pathologies.

Though nobody within the Unit managed to firmly locate themselves within the dissenting enclave position of low grid/ high group, it is interesting to note how some staff otherwise escaped from or were cast out of the bureaucratic high grid/ high group position that most staff occupied. Doctors and managers, as experts, gravitated towards a low grid/low group individual position, though some became discredited and fell from grace into the high grid/low group isolate position. Low status nurses gravitated towards this isolate position. From their respective places within the grid/group map, they often held unsympathetic and antagonistic views of those located elsewhere.

Individuals (risk takers): Although, as the most dominant professional within health care, medics can operate a high degree of autonomy, as Freidson points out (1970), professional autonomy is always relative. The Home Office considerably regulates forensic psychiatrists' treatment of patients through the operation of mental health care legislation. However, despite this constraint, the forensic psychiatrists in this study emphasised their autonomy, expert knowledge and leadership within MDTs. Their high level of symbolic capital was particularly apparent in the MDT workshop as the non-medical staff (mostly nurses) responded to our question of 'what enables MDT practice to succeed?' A number of staff told us, very deferentially, that this depended on whether the consultant would allow it.

The consultants conveyed an image of being able to control and manage the dangers, through their own expertise, that their clients posed rather than through the bureaucratic controls of the organisation. This was particularly apparent at a seminar in which a nurse (Timothy) stated that nurses were unable to initiate therapeutic activities with clients on the ward because of staff shortages, which limited them to custodial duties. A psychiatrist (Helena) responded, declaring that whenever she visited the wards, nurses were far from busy, frequently reading newspapers. By contrast, she boasted that she was able to run therapeutic groups by herself, with a dozen clients who might well act in a dangerous manner. Psychiatrists were seemingly more confident in their professional ability to take risks.

Some nurses complained that psychiatrists took risks recklessly in admitting patients to the Unit. As Nurse Manager Norman explained:

> Consultants are bringing in people, responding to emergencies but not really thinking like: 'What, wait a minute, you've got three or four with very complex character individuals' which I worry about in units like this ... I'd stopped one consultant bringing one patient in. This was a man who was on what we call a 'three man lock'. In other words, he was specialised all the time by three prison officers. We had one of them in two days before that, and they wanted to bring him in for the same week. And I said: 'No, you have got to give us three or four days until we get this person settled before we can have the next one'. But that's the concern that I have here, and I feel that these consultants don't want to know. They want their patient in, in their time and they're not interested in other people. (Nurse Manager Norman, individual general interview)

Expertise and leadership were also claimed by a succession of managers, such as the nurse manager quoted above, who offers an account of himself heroically challenging a psychiatrist. In the three years of our study there were numerous changes in staff personnel, with each new manager boasting that s/he would sweep away the inefficiencies of the past. The ward nurses were often cynical of such management. As a ward manager said

> management here is like a tide, it comes and goes out and we have almost three-monthly tides ... /. ... Since I have been here I have had five different managers in two years, yeah, and I have had five different opinions which I have to implement, so there is inconsistency. (Ward manager Beverley, individual general interview)

Staff at ward level did not always regard the actions of leaders positively. In the MDT workshop, an OT, Tanya, attempted to define what hindered successful MDT working. She explained that successful MDT working and good patient care were achieved by determined and inconspicuous care co-ordination. However, such work achieved little recognition within the organisation. Rather, she suggested, 'leaders and saboteurs' got noticed and that a synergy existed between the two. Rather contradictorily, the main staff group displayed considerable deference towards the organisation's medical experts, rarely disagreeing with them, whilst seemingly wanting greater equality with them. Psychiatrists, managers and others in a leadership role were seemingly concerned to demonstrate their value to the organisation as experts by initiating change that was noticed by others. If they failed to do so they ran the risk of being identified as ineffectual. Therefore, they engaged in ambitious risk taking. However, some staff saw these experts as a destructive nuisance rather than as entrepreneurial developers of the organisation.

Isolate (risk enduring and creative exploitation): Living under lock and key and regulated by staff, the patients, often alone in their view of themselves and the world around them, were most certainly in the isolate position. However, two types of people amongst the staff group also gravitated towards the isolate position. These were first, discredited managers, and second, unqualified staff and junior nurses, both of whom were on the margins of the staff group. Both patients and staff in this high grid/low group position expressed frustration about their lack of control within the organisation. As previously described by a charge nurse, managers were carried in and out on a management tide that swept through the Unit every so often. Whilst on the in-coming tide these managers boasted to us in interview of the changes they would make, presenting an image of being able to supply the Unit with their expertise. Yet, once they became discredited they were swept from the position of individual expert to that of isolate, expelled on an outward tide from the Unit. Out at sea they were lost to our study. However, one nurse manager, whose controversial reporting of a SUI was shortly followed by his departure, told us that he had experienced hostility from other staff and received anonymous threatening phone calls.

Meanwhile, high grid/low group staff, at the lower end of the organisational hierarchy, saw themselves as excluded from the decision-making procedures of its bureaucracy. A health care assistant attending the MDT workshop conveyed this sentiment as he explained that he had come to the workshop to learn about what went on 'in meetings behind locked doors'. Nursing staff expressed fatalistic resignation about being unsupported within the organisation, which often left them exposed to risk. Illustrative stories were told to us of how patients were able to attack and injure nurses with impunity. Furthermore, some staff described how control was lost in the management of patients. One nurse explained the situation on his ward as follows:

> Staff in general who are accustomed to work in rehab, taking patients on trips, taking patients home to their family, taking them shopping; they have never dealt with acutely ill females and they're scared! We have had incidents on the ward where the staff are so terrified that they can't even pull the alarm and in my opinion that's unsafe, but that's what's going on. (Charge Nurse, Kunle, individual general interview)

The staff in lower positions within the hierarchy felt less power to control the risks they faced in their work environment. Nurses repeatedly stated that they were 'there twenty-four/seven with the patients' and were, therefore, not only more exposed to risk but also had particularly valuable insights into the patients' risk potential. Some unqualified nursing staff proposed that their claim to this insightful position was far stronger than that of their trained colleagues who often extricated themselves from the ward in office duties and meetings. Greater exposure to contact with patients was associated with both a greater exposure to their potentially violent behaviour and a greater awareness of patients' day-to-day behaviour and thinking. One unqualified nurse spoke of how this close contact with patients made her acutely aware of the potential danger that patients posed, which she thought went unacknowledged by trained nurses, who failed to take notice of her concerns about the danger she recognised in patients.

The staff at the lower end of the organisational hierarchy regarded themselves as practically excluded from a bureaucracy within which they wished to have a greater stake. They therefore felt themselves to be a 'done to' group of people exposed to risk that they had little power to control. Patients also understood themselves as a done to group, though in more extreme terms, as they felt far more alienated by the bureaucracy. Held in a locked environment, subject to rules and continual judgement about their behaviour they were, undoubtedly, in a higher grid position than high grid staff. Service users spoke about being exposed to risks that they were powerless to control. They spoke of having to take medicine that some perceived as doing them more harm than good, being convicted of crimes they did not commit or had been provoked into committing, having their children taken away from them and other such misfortunes. They spoke of how their lives were slipping away from them and how they feared becoming institutionalised within the Unit and within the forensic psychiatric system of which the Unit was a part.

Though the patients considered themselves to be victims of unfair and unhelpful treatment, having endured and currently enduring considerable risks, the staff (like the core of the city they were charged with protecting) primarily regarded the patients as a source of danger. Like homosexuals, drug addicts and prostitutes within the city dealing with the threat of AIDS, they were regarded as the 'at risk' group, in need of control. The central community of the city employs similar means to deal with both the threat of AIDS and deinstitutionalised madness. In both instances, health care professionals are recruited to teach 'at risk' groups how to control the threat they pose to society. It was highly apparent within staff interviews that they regarded the development of insight amongst patients as a major objective of their work. As Douglas (1992) points out, the central community is quite sure that it is right and that opposing views and perspectives from its fringes are wrong. It therefore regards education (or therapy) as the only way to deal with opposition from 'benighted' people at the margins of society. Some of the patients we spoke to appeared to have realised that they needed to be successfully educated (or 'converted', as Goffman (1961) terms it) in order to make progress. As one patient said of his group therapy:

> The nurse told us [a group of patients in therapy] quite frankly that this is the gateway, the doorway to freedom. You know. That's what she said. And I appreciated that, you know. Afterwards I thought it was fantastic that she said that. I never heard anybody else say it before, you know ... / ... . Yeah, I can pay attention to things better than what I used to. I can see better, you know. That's what I told them in classes [group therapy sessions], you know. (Patient Tom, individual case study interview)

Yet, as some of the practitioners we spoke to realised, people have understandable reasons, not simply to do with their ignorance for resisting the education/therapy they were offered. As a psychiatrist explained:

> I despair when people think patients should just easily develop insight. I mean if I've had a row with my boyfriend, then it takes an awful lot for me to admit that I am wrong. And we expect these people who are often of low IQ and low social class to readily admit to the major things they have done, like killing their children. (Medical Consultant Helena, at a seminar)

Resisting education/therapy was also one of many ways in which patients confounded the system. As we have seen, staff commonly recognised that patients often sabotaged their progress, and that particular types of patients were thought to subvert the functioning of the organisation. Subversion was sometimes done in highly elaborate ways. For example, in interview, a psychologist explained how a patient [Boyd] admitted committing serious crimes, leading to a police investigation, which proved Boyd's claim to be a complete fabrication. Patient Boyd's psychologist, somewhat humiliated by the experience, explained that this patient regularly indulged in such 'cat and mouse games' with him. Staff could and did explain such behaviour as symptomatic of patients' pathologies. For example, in a case review meeting for Boyd a doctor suggested to the psychologist that the patient's game playing was a form of sadism, symptomatic of the patient's personality disorder. However, such behaviour could also be regarded as the response of an isolate to his marginalisation in the high grid/low group position. For, as Douglas points out, though isolates are largely ineffectual 'disorganized as they are ... they can often find ways of exploiting the rest of the system, for creativity and even financial gain' (1992:106). Patient Boyd appeared to be highly sucessful in creatively manipulating the system that had deprived him of his autonomy.

Figure 5.2, summarises the four ideal type position of the grid/group analysis of the Unit that we have outlined above. Before concluding this chapter we offer some reflexive thoughts about our own position in the Unit in relation to our grid/group analysis.

Position of researchers (experts, dissenters and isolates): The staff of the Unit granted us access as we academics proclaimed expertise to be able to produce knowledge that they might find useful. At times, we are arrogant enough to believe this grandiose claim of ours and that this chapter and other writing emanating from this research project (Heyman *et al.* 2004) might be of interest to fellow academics. We represent our place in the map (see Figure 5.2) in the expert, dissenter and isolate positions (parenthesis indicating our minimal significance, at least to staff). We found ourselves, at various times, partially in all of these positions in the course of our study as we skirted around the edge of the staff group.

Perhaps the best description of how we seemed to be regarded by the staff of the Unit was as dubious experts, of uncertain identity and trustworthiness. There was some interest amongst the staff in our research and in the academic expertise we claimed to offer. Between ten to twenty staff attended seminars and meetings each time we presented our findings on five different occasions. Yet what was particularly striking to us, was how forgettable we were to many of them. Repeated introduction of ourselves and explanations of our research project was, seemingly, not committed to the memory of a number of staff that repeatedly queried who we were.

However, we were noticed as a potential danger and even an external threat to the staff on several occasions. When we gave a verbal account of our findings at a staff seminar two psychiatrists questioned the objectivity and trustworthiness of our research. They attempted to discredit our research for not having a clear hypothesis and expressed fear and anger that we might publish 'unscientific', untruthful and negative reports about the Unit, which would have repercussions on them. It was as though we had emerged as a dissenting enclave, threatening the Unit's knowledge base.

On another occasion, when the principal investigator for this research visited a ward to interview a patient, a nurse insisted on searching the researcher's bag for illicit drugs and escape tools. Though two of us were given formal introductory security training to allow us an electronic key with which we could move through the Unit, this privilege was withdrawn towards the end of our research as our training was declared expired. This situation arose when we introduced ourselves to a medical secretary, as we attempted to recruit people to the MDT workshop. Unable to convey to her who we were and what our mission was (despite valiant attempts) we left and visited a ward that we had been to many times before. The secretary soon after phoned the ward to instruct the nurse to escort us off the premises immediately. Somewhat embarrassed, the nurse politely complied with the secretary's order and we left, having been identified as an alien threat that needed to be expelled. We joked with each other about the 'Alice in Wonderland' type experience we had of the Unit's organisational bureaucracy. However, what our experience does illustrate is how uncomfortable and alienating it can feel to be an outsider within a secure unit, which can prove a monumental and hostile force. We had not established a strong enough bond of alliance with its staff to achieve the comfortable respected position of experts. The staff only minimally valued our knowledge and insights. Yet our position was a lot more comfortable than that of the isolates within the Unit to whom we spoke. Like us, they expressed frustration with the rulings of bureaucrats who understood them as deviants and a threat to the integrity of the organisation. As Douglas (1992) tells us bureaucrats, from their high/grid high/group position, are typically 'clogged' yet 'smug'. However, our fate was very different from that of the patients. The staff could, at worst, only banish us from their citadel. Such isolation was far more preferable to the fate of the patients who were captive within it.

Conclusion

Our experience is, of course, a product of our chosen methodology, which entailed a marginal presence and involvement with the Unit. This is not ideal for the cultural analysis that we have attempted to develop in this chapter. Ideally, we would have been able to more comprehensively compare talk with action, to understand more fully how individuals experienced, thought about and dealt with risk. However, over three years, we were able to piece together a substantial amount of observational data from a variety of sources towards an analysis that has not just relied upon talk.

The application of Douglas's grid/group model has proved useful in understanding how the staff of a forensic mental health care unit shaped its culture, and how that culture shaped their risk thinking and actions. We have seen how this model can produce an analysis that is far from static, for we have seen how, even within a highly regulated organisation, people influence and change their position and that of others. The model should not be understood as defining four actual places at the four corners of a map, but relative cultural positions towards which people with greater power move themselves and others, whilst those with lesser power become positioned. As our reflective consideration of our own position within the Unit has shown, actors within the system are best understood as being somewhere indefinitely within the map, at times migrating from or being pushed from one position to another.

Actors in these various positions of grid and group often seemed to be oblivious or intolerant of the risk experience and thinking of those in other positions, as they blamed each other. Though our analysis explains how a plurality of risk thinking and action is socially produced within a forensic mental health care secure unit, we suggest that similarities may be found not just in other secure units but also in other health care institutions managing other risks. We suggest that this analysis offers a chance for nurses (as the main readers of this book) and others within other health care organisations that manage risk, to consider how culture affects their risk thinking and actions and that of others.

6 The very LOUD discourses of risk in pregnancy

*Karen MacKinnon
and Liza McCoy*

Introduction

This chapter draws on the work of Dorothy Smith (1987, 1999) to develop a feminist analysis of the way discourses of risk operate in the lives of childbearing women and the nurses who work with them. Although pregnancy is a healthy state, it has long been associated with a range of risks and dangers. In wealthy societies, the locus of concern is the baby rather than the mother, as maternal deaths in childbirth are rare. Preterm birth is identified as the most important cause of infant mortality and morbidity in industrialised countries such as Canada (Canadian Perinatal Surveillance System 2003). This chapter focuses on discourses of risk for preterm birth and the operation of a preterm birth prevention project in one Canadian city, examined from the standpoint of women experiencing preterm labour.

Recent policy changes that shift the care for women experiencing preterm labour from the hospital to the home, have restructured responsibility for preventing preterm birth from the institution to the individual woman and family. Individualising risk discourses thus intersect with economic and social discourses that locate responsibility for caring work in the 'private' sphere, while rendering invisible the actual conditions of women's lives. Women's employment and caregiving work fall outside the narrow biomedical risk frame; they

are not formally recognised as sources of risk, nor
the conditions under which women experiencii
labour carry out their work of 'keeping the bal
result is a risk discourse around preterm birth that
a form of social control over pregnant women, promoting an
overwhelming sense of personal responsibility for preventing
preterm birth and, for some women, fear, guilt and shame.

Reconceiving preterm labour in the restructured Canadian context

Health care in Canada is funded by transfer payments from the
federal government to the ten provinces. Although the 1984
Canada Health Act establishes national standards of universal
coverage, health care is a provincial jurisdiction and each
provincial government is responsible for administering its own
system of health insurance and health service delivery. In the
early 1990s, health care transfer payments were reduced when
the Canadian government adopted a policy of fiscal restraint
that involved cutting social spending in order to shrink and
eventually eliminate the national financial deficit. Some
provincial governments also pursued their own policies of fiscal
restraint, and the combined effect on health care delivery was
significant. Health administrators sought ways to streamline
health services and make them more efficient through the
introduction of business management techniques. Services
were trimmed, staff laid off, waiting times increased, hospitals
closed beds, and many responsibilities for health care were
transferred to the 'community' (read: women, the unpaid
caregivers). As Neysmith noted: 'there is very little recognition
of how restructuring increases and changes the caring labour
that women do and how these get played out in gendered,
classed, and racialized ways' (2000: 1).

Childbearing women most often receive prenatal care from
community-based physicians with postnatal care supplemented
by home visits from public health nurses. Although midwives
have recently re-entered the Canadian health care system as
community-based practitioners, most Canadian women give
birth in hospitals, assisted by nurses and doctors. Between 1990

and 2000 restructured maternity services resulted in an increase in early postpartum discharge, and postpartum hospital stays for Canadian women decreased from 3.6 days to 2.4 days following vaginal birth. By 2001, women in the province of Alberta were discharged earlier than women in all the other Canadian provinces following both vaginal and cesarean delivery (Canadian Perinatal Surveillance System 2003).

The widespread restructuring of health services in Canada took place at the same time as developments in computer technology, enabled epidemiologists and public health specialists to create institutionalised health surveillance systems. One such system, the Canadian Perinatal Surveillance System (CPSS), was formalised in 1995; the first Canadian Perinatal Health Report was published in 2000 (CPSS 2003). The CPSS facilitates the tracking and comparison of 27 perinatal health indicators, including preterm birth rates across provinces and nationally. In Canada, the preterm birth rate has been increasing. By the year 2000, the preterm birth rate in Canada had increased to 7.6 per cent of live births from 6.6 per cent in 1991. Potential explanations for this increase include increased rates of obstetrical intervention for the compromised fetus, increased multiple birth rates due to reproductive technologies, and more complete registration of early gestation live births (CPSS 2003). Although these explanations point to medical 'advances', the care of fragile preterm infants in Neonatal Intensive Care Units nonetheless represents a significant health service expenditure.

In this context of rising health costs and health services restructuring, the Canadian Preterm Birth Consensus Conference was held (Niday and Kinch 1998). The 'consensus' generated by participants recommended a shift from identifying high-risk women to primary and secondary prevention, since identifiable risk factors have only been found for about half of the women who deliver prematurely (Heaman *et al.* 2001; Stewart 1998). Many health care providers believed that earlier identification of preterm labour might lead to improved birth outcomes. Recommendations included warning *all* pregnant women about the dangers of preterm birth and teaching them to recognise the symptoms of early preterm labour and report these to their caregivers.

In Alberta, regional preterm birth prevention programmes were developed that implemented the recommendations of the Preterm Birth Consensus Conference. In Calgary, an Alberta city with a population of just under one million people, all pregnant women were targeted in a programme that included large advertisement panels on the exterior of city buses, warning that: 'If you are pregnant, then preterm labour can happen to you!' Patient education materials were developed for distribution at prenatal classes and by health providers. Among the symptoms the new materials asked pregnant women to report to their caregivers were painful or painless uterine contractions. Prior to this time, contractions during pregnancy were referred to as Braxton Hicks contractions and considered by health professionals to be part of the normal childbearing experience. Today, uterine contractions have been reconstructed as a symptom of preterm labour.

Preterm labour is an uncertain diagnosis (Steven-Simon and Orleans 1999) based on ambiguous symptoms (Weiss *et al.* 2002), with little effective treatment (Enkin and Keirse 2000). Current medical treatment for preterm labour (including bed rest) has not been shown to reduce the risk of preterm birth (Goldenberg and Rouse 1998), and the 'stubborn challenge of preterm birth' remains (Lumley 2003). A decade ago most Canadian women diagnosed with preterm labour were cared for in hospital settings by perinatal nurses and physicians. With the shift to community-based care, more pregnant women are sent home to live alongside the 'threat' of preterm labour. Antenatal home care programmes have been developed to assist some of these women and provide ongoing health surveillance of them and their unborn babies. But for the most part, the responsibility for prevention and the burden of care has been transferred to women and their families.

The research – exploring the social organisation of women's preterm labour experiences

Institutional ethnography is a method of inquiry developed by Dorothy Smith (1987, 1999, 2001, 2002) as a way to realise the project of a feminist sociology *for* people. As Smith explains

'Institutional ethnography takes up a stance in people's experience in the local sites of their bodily being and seeks to discover what can't be grasped from within that experience, namely the social relations that are implicit in its organization' (2001: 161) (see also Campbell and Gregor 2002; DeVault and McCoy 2002). The goal is not to explain people's behaviour but to explicate the institutional relations of power in which people's lives are embedded. Institutional ethnographic research, therefore, usually starts in the embodied experience of some group of people and investigates how that experience takes shape within a particular set of institutional and discursive relations.

The concept of discourse used in institutional ethnography draws on Foucault's notion of discourse but 'stretch[es] it in ways that escape Foucault's paradigm' (Smith 2002: 41):

> we want to address discourse as a conversation mediated by texts that is not a matter of statements alone but of actual ongoing practices and sites of practices, the material forms of texts (journals, reviews, books, conferences, classrooms, laboratories, etc.), the methods of producing texts. ... Texts are understood as embedded in and organizing relations among subjects active in the discourse. We are talking then about actual people entering into actual relations with one another. (Smith 1987: 214)

Institutional ethnography has been taken up by a number of researchers investigating the institutional and discursive field of health care and the embodied experience of people who participate in those relations. Campbell (1998, 2001) studied the training of nurses and the restructuring of nurses' work. Rankin (2001) discovered how nurses were pulled into doing 'the fiscal work of health care reform' as the texts they used to document their work imported a business logic into the everyday practices of a hospital setting. Mykhalovskiy showed how 'care pathway' texts have been used to 'standardize and reduce the duration of care provided to heart attack patients' (2001: 269). Other institutional ethnographies have studied nursing homes (Diamond 1992) and a psychiatric day programme (Townsend 1998), from an entry point in the experience of front-line health care workers. Institutional ethnography has also been used to examine health care and home care services from the standpoint of patients and clients (Campbell *et al.* 1998; Mykhalovskiy and McCoy 2002).

This chapter offers a first report from an institutional ethnographic study into the social organisation of women's preterm labour experiences. The first author of this chapter, Karen MacKinnon, recruited and interviewed eight women who all self-identified as having experienced preterm labour in the past five months. Interviews focused on the women's experiences of learning about the risk of preterm labour and living with preterm labour as well as the work they did caring for themselves, their unborn babies and their families. Four of the women delivered a preterm baby within two weeks of experiencing preterm labour symptoms. The other four women first experienced preterm labour between 24 and 34 weeks of their most recent pregnancy, lived alongside the 'threat' of preterm labour for the rest of their pregnancy, and gave birth to a healthy full term baby. Within the framework of institutional ethnography, these eight women do not constitute a 'sample'; rather they serve as a panel of expert informants 'whose experience generates the problematic to be investigated and provides the entry point into a set of institutional relations' (McCoy, in press).

Following up on the interview conversations, Karen conducted naturalistic observation in hospital settings, since it is to hospitals that women go when they experience what might be preterm labour. She observed nursing work in three labour and delivery triage settings (where women were first assessed when they came to the hospital) as well as nurses' work on antepartum in-patient units. Chart forms and other institutional texts were examined in their context of use. Karen also reflected on her own understandings of the community context for care from her work as a Community Health Nurse working in an antenatal home care programme for women experiencing pregnancy complications.

The discussion that follows examines how, in Calgary, Alberta, the risks of preterm birth are conceptualised and promoted in distinctively individualising ways. The focus is on how pregnant women are enlisted into this risk discourse and how the terms of the discourse organise the hospital setting and the work of nurses and other health care providers.

Enlisting women in the risk discourse: The work of the Preterm Birth Prevention Text

One woman, Katrina,[1] remembered being given a hand-out on preterm labour by her nurse at her 26 week routine prenatal visit.

> *Katrina:* And she says, she says that at the twenty-six week point we give this to people to, just *because it can happen* basically.
>
> *Karen M.:* Right.
>
> *Katrina:* And you know they want *you* to be aware of what can happen and ...
>
> *Karen M.:* Okay.
>
> *Katrina:* how to prevent it and, or as much as *you* possibly can.

Texts are more than passive transmitters of content or meaning. Dorothy Smith suggests that they are active like speakers in a conversation: 'active in "speaking" to us as our reading activates them' (1999: 135). Katrina was talking about receiving a local health region document written for the Preterm Birth Prevention Program. This institutional text is available in two forms: as a glossy 'tear-off' sheet, designed to be handed out by health care providers in a variety of settings, and as a section integrated into a spiral bound book called *From Here Through Maternity* (Calgary Health Region 2001)[2] published especially for women in the health region. A lot of care and attention has gone into the selection of materials for this book, which was designed to replace a myriad of pamphlets that childbearing families inevitably lost. This text suggests that *all* pregnant women are *at risk* for preterm labour and birth. 'Signs of preterm labour should never be ignored. Half of all preterm births occur to women with no known risk factors' (Calgary Health Region 2001: 38). The original tear-off shet uses capital letters for emphasis as follows: 'What YOU SHOULD DO if YOU have SIGNS of preterm labour' (Calgary Health Region 1999: 38). Women are instructed to

---

[1] The names used to identify women are the pseudonyms that they selected.

[2] The Calgary Health Region adapted materials that were developed in another Canadian province, so this type of preterm birth prevention text may not be unique to Calgary. These patient education materials are currently being revised.

call their doctor or midwife right away. Signs of preterm labour are formulated as follows:

Some women just know that something is not right, but specific signs include

- contractions (may be painful or painless)
- cramps (may feel like menstrual cramps or gas pains)
- fluid gush or leak of fluid from the vagina
- change or increase in vaginal discharge
- bleeding from the vagina
- changes in low back pain
- full or heavy feeling in vagina. (Calgary Health Region 2001: 38)

The early signs of preterm labour are subtle and ambiguous (Weis *et al.* 2002). Although most Canadian women probably know that vaginal bleeding during pregnancy is not normal, the rest of these symptoms are hard to differentiate from normal pregnancy changes. Learning to sort out which contractions or other symptoms to pay attention to has become part of the work of learning to live alongside the threat of preterm labour.

The next section is entitled 'How You Can Reduce the risk factors' and the suggested actions include 'stop smoking, avoid alcohol and drugs, avoid all injuries, seek prenatal care early in pregnancy and choose a healthy lifestyle' (Calgary Health Region 2001: 38). This list formulates risk factors as under the control, and therefore the responsibility of, individual pregnant women. Even the hazards of living or the actions of other people, such as abusive partners or bad drivers, are implicitly produced as the woman's action and responsibility when women are advised to 'avoid all injury' in order to prevent preterm birth. The advice to 'choose a healthy lifestyle' further individualises risk and discounts the context of women's lives. Most women living in poverty do not choose this 'lifestyle'.

This patient education material asks women to monitor their bodies without reference to the context of their lives. Women who are working or who are busy caring for preschool children may not have the opportunity to practise the kind of diligent self-surveillance required to detect subtle signs of preterm labour. This decontextualised medical advice, then, has the potential to increase guilt for some childbearing women who miss or ignore these early non-specific signs. Other women are likely to become more diligent as a result of this discourse, sometimes in ways that may not make much difference in birth outcome but cast a shadow of guilt and worry over their pregnancy experience.

This text designates the woman as responsible for avoiding risks to her pregnancy, practising self-surveillance to identify, in a timely way, early signs of preterm labour, presenting herself to medical authority, and by implication, complying with medical treatment recommendations, which can include hospitalisation but almost always includes quitting work and staying home on bed rest. This version of the woman as responsible is only effective, however, if women take up this discourse. Katrina took up this text by paying more attention to her body's cues. At 34 weeks she experienced three very strong contractions over a two-hour period. Using the textual information provided she recognised that these contractions were 'not normal' so she called the local telehealth[3] phone line. It is important to remember that in the past, consulting different resource material, Katrina might have recognised these symptoms as normal Braxton Hicks contractions. Following the advice of the nurse on the telephone, she and her partner went to the hospital for assessment. Let us, for the moment, leave Katrina and her partner on their way to the hospital and pause to consider what *isn't* mentioned in the educational material on preterm birth prevention.

Absent discourses

Another way of analysing the activity of a text is to think carefully about what is not said. Texts create patterns of visibility and invisibility; they provide for what can be known and represent states of affairs in ways that render them institutionally actionable. When the Calgary materials are read alongside other accounts of preterm birth prevention, and in relation to other preterm birth prevention strategies, some striking omissions come into view.

---

[3] The telehealth phone line described would be similar to NHS Direct in the Great Britain.

Occupational or work-related stress has been investigated as a source of risk for preterm birth (Bodin *et al.* 1999), and evidence suggests a link between rates of preterm birth and the working conditions of pregnant women. Mozurkewich *et al.* (2000) conducted a meta-analysis that showed that working conditions may influence preterm birth rates. Significant positive associations were found between preterm birth and physically demanding work, work that involved prolonged standing, work with high work fatigue scores, and shift work. A Canadian study conducted in Quebec City found that standing at work for more than two hours and psychosocial stressors (family illness, mortality, disruption, violence or financial distress) were risk factors for preterm birth (Moutquin 2003). France has been described as a natural experiment in preterm birth prevention. When a nationally funded programme of prenatal care and early (before 28 weeks) work-leave was implemented in the early 1970s, rates of spontaneous preterm births decreased from 6.92 per cent in 1972 to 3.8 per cent in 1988/1989 (Papiernik 1999). Sweden has similar low rates of preterm birth and well-developed social programmes that may play a role in preterm birth prevention. In Sweden researchers have developed a semi-structured work history interview for care providers to assess the need for job adjustment in pregnancy (Wergeland and Strand 1998). A recent European study of employment, working conditions, and preterm birth attempted to take the social and legislative context of women's pregnancy experiences into consideration (Saurel-Cubizolles *et al.* 2004). These researchers concluded that specific working conditions affect the risk of preterm birth and that employment-related risks could be mediated by 'social policies granting women paid leaves in pregnancy and limiting exposures to onerous working conditions in pregnancy' (Saurel-Cubizolles *et al.* 2004: 395).

Perhaps not surprisingly in a politically conservative, 'employer-friendly' province, work-related risks have been noticeably absent from the local information provided as part of the preterm birth prevention programme.[4] The absence

---

[4] The 2004 edition of *From Here Through Maternity* is expected to include some information about employment and pregnancy.

of advice related to working conditions in these education materials is particularly striking because a nationally distributed book, produced by the Society of Obstetricians and Gynaecologists of Canada (2000: 39), does include working long hours (more than eight hours per day), shift work, and physically strenuous work in the list of risk factors for premature birth. It also offers a checklist to help pregnant women determine if their job is strenuous (2000: 45). Pregnant women in Calgary, however, are not given enough information to decide whether they should continue working into the second and third trimester of pregnancy.

In Calgary, employment does not enter into the preterm birth prevention discourse until women have experienced symptoms of preterm labour and are told to stop working. This contrasts with the primary prevention approach in many European countries that rely on job assessments and early work leaves to reduce preterm births. These countries have developed an understanding of risk as socially generated; the burden of cost and effort for minimising risk is spread out, borne partly by employers and taxpayers. In Alberta, employers are not recruited into the risk discourse, which remains highly individualised and focused on the responsibility and self-surveillance of pregnant women.

Working women in Canada are entitled to maternity leave (15 weeks) and parental leave benefits (35 weeks) under the national Employment Insurance benefits program. Women can choose to take maternity leave up to 12 weeks before their due date but can only collect maternity benefits eight weeks before they are 'due' unless they are prescribed to be off work for medical reasons (Government of Alberta 2004). Women who begin their paid leave during pregnancy will have less time at home with their baby after the baby is born. Most of the women interviewed for this study had planned to work as long as possible during their pregnancy. Several women also verbalised a competing discourse of saving Employment Insurance benefits for 'after the baby comes'. What we can see is how the legislative framework, combined with various risk discourses (risk to pregnancy, risk to child of poor mother-child bonding, risk of not breastfeeding long enough), puts the onus on women and leaves them in a double-bind situation.

They can take early leave and possibly prevent preterm labour, but at the cost of giving up important bonding and breast-feeding time with the baby.

What happens when a woman comes into the hospital setting

We left Katrina and her partner on the way to the hospital to have her symptoms of preterm labour assessed. In Calgary women who think they are having signs of preterm labour might call their doctor's office or a telephone help line operated by the Health Region, or they might call the hospital directly and be put through to a nurse working on the Labour and Delivery Triage area. No matter which of these sites the woman calls, she will most likely be told to go to the hospital for assessment. Nurses working in this area frequently talked about 'not taking chances' and 'covering yourself,' reflecting the power of current risk management discourses. When giving telephone advice to childbearing women, nurses at the hospital almost always said: 'come in to be checked just in case'. This 'covering yourself' response speaks to the degree of fear perinatal nurses working in this setting experienced related to perceived legal risks. There is, however, a tension between telling almost all women to 'come in for assessment' and the extra traffic this strategy generates in the triage unit, which increases the stress on nurses within an already-busy health care system. (There is as yet no statistical data to show that preterm labour assessments are causing an increase in triage visits, although anecdotal evidence suggests this may indeed be the case.[5])

Obstetrical triage units are relatively new institutional structures in Canada (MacDonald *et al.* 1993). They were initially designed to provide an opportunity to assess women quickly, to avoid admitting women too early in labour, and to avoid unnecessary institutional work processes associated with hospital admission. The triage units observed were very busy places. After arriving, women were initially assessed by an experienced Labour and Delivery nurse. This nurse would rapidly assess

[5] The Calgary Health Region has recently begun collecting this kind of data. (M. Quance, 2004, personal communication).

the seriousness of the situation and was responsible for ensuring that those (few) women who needed to see a physician immediately did so. She would also hook the woman up to a fetal monitor, so that her contractions could be 'objectively' confirmed, and begin to complete the 'Maternity Triage' form. Bed pressures and nurses' rationing work were clearly demonstrated during these triage observations. Declining numbers of primary care providers for childbearing women in Calgary have resulted in triage units operating as walk-in clinics for pregnant women. There are also a limited number of hospital beds available for admitting women, so triage functions as a 'holding tank' for women waiting for a bed. Also, women seen in triage are required to be checked by a 'responsible' physician before leaving (unless they leave against medical advice), which results in many women waiting for long periods to be seen by the designated physician who has many competing priorities.

Medical triage refers to the screening of patients or casualties into three groups to determine the relative priority for treatment (see: Stedman's Medical Dictionary (Hensyl 1990: 1628)). Observations in triage showed how women who came to the hospital with symptoms of preterm labour were sorted into three groups based on how likely they were to deliver a preterm baby. One group was labelled by nurses as 'active' and were the most likely women to receive a medical diagnosis of preterm labour. Another group had symptoms that fitted biomedical constructions of preterm labour but their contractions had 'settled' without changing their cervix. These women received a diagnosis of 'threatened preterm labour' and included women who experienced symptoms that were on the list given out by the preterm birth prevention programme. Some of these women had experienced periods of painful uterine contractions the night before they came into triage for assessment. The third group of women came in with symptoms that either didn't fit biomedical constructions of preterm labour or their symptoms were seen by experienced labour and delivery nurses as part of the normal pregnancy experience.

Women whose symptoms of preterm labour were confirmed, either by the presence of active contractions or changes to the woman's cervix over a two-hour time span, were diagnosed with preterm labour and usually admitted to the hospital for at least 24 hours. Medical treatment included the administration of indomethacin and/or morphine to help stop labour (this treatment has been shown to postpone labour for 48 hours) and the administration of steroids to help the baby's lungs mature. Women were closely monitored for contractions, put on bed rest with bathroom privileges, their urine was checked for infection and they might receive intravenous fluids for the treatment of dehydration if this was a suspected cause for their preterm labour episode. If their symptoms 'settled' and their baby was not born at this time, the women were discharged and usually prescribed bed rest at home.

Most of the women observed during the eight days of triage observations were sorted into one or other of the 'non-active' groups. The preterm birth prevention discourse enlists women to pay attention to their bodily cues and call the hospital or telephone help line if they have any concerns that 'something is not right'. A nurse, Kathy, suggested that over-diligence might be one effect of the preterm birth prevention programme. She said that most women who come in for assessment of preterm labour do not have active symptoms or changes to their cervix. Given the institutional work processes routinely required for assessment of the woman's symptoms and the work-up of risk, it is easy to understand how busy nurses get frustrated when many women come in with cramping, mild contractions or 'leaking' that rarely progresses to preterm birth. In addition, obstetrical triage was organised by unit priorities and discourses of efficiency and cost effectiveness, with a focus on dealing with the problem and getting the women out or 'clearing triage'.

Katrina went to the hospital for assessment three times during her pregnancy, first because she experienced some strong contractions and later for leaking watery fluid. She sensed that one of the nurses didn't think she needed to be there, although she had been told by her physician to come back if she had any concerns.

> *Katrina:* No, the nurses, I found the nurses there were very, especially the one that first received me and brought me in. She was very like, 'ah'[loud exhale], like annoyed almost.
>
> *Karen M.:* Okay, okay.
>
> *Katrina:* You know and I understand ...

Karen M.: She made you feel like you were, shouldn't have come in, did she?

Katrina: A little bit, like she didn't say it but just her attitude and when you'd ask her a question, it was kind of like, 'Oh God, are you that stupid?' You know, that's almost what you got from her.

Katrina was also 34 weeks gestation when she first experienced symptoms of preterm labour. Although preterm labour is defined as 'labour that occurs too early' or 'more than 3 weeks before your due date' (Calgary Health Region 2001: 38), health care providers did not seem overly concerned after the woman reached 34 weeks. At the triage unit, nurses explained that medical management was no different from normal child-birth at this point and that nothing was likely to be done to stop the woman from having her baby. This discrepancy in the time frame requiring diligent watching is troubling, especially since contractions are much more common after 34 weeks of pregnancy. Women may be conscripted into continuing their health surveillance work when it is no longer required or appreciated by medical personnel. Katrina's blood pressure increased late in her pregnancy so her labour was induced. She gave birth to a healthy full-term baby girl.

Biomedical focus on individualised risk

A great deal of the work in triage involved the repetitive assessment of 'risk factors' and the completion of institutional forms and procedures. What is, perhaps, most striking is that the same questions were asked repeatedly by a variety of health care personnel. Women were asked questions about risks before pregnancy (such as age, weight, medical conditions), risks from their past obstetrical history (such as preterm birth, small for dates babies and other pregnancy complications), risks experienced during their current pregnancy (such as antepartum bleeding or previous hospitalisations), and risks seen as relevant to their presenting concern (e.g., menstrual cramps, contractions, leaking fluid). Both the nurses and the women observed in this setting expressed their frustration with asking or answering the same questions over and over again. One effect of this repetitive assessment of risk factors might have been to impress women with the seriousness of their situation, enhancing the likelihood they would strive to comply with the medical treatment plan.

As the only hospital employee consistently present in triage, the nurse also worked through her charting to protect the hospital from legal risks. Charting consumed significant amounts of nursing time but was seen by nurses as very important in this setting to 'protect yourself' from legal risk. When doctors and hospitals in the highly litigious field of obstetrics are able to demonstrate that they have done everything possible, their legal position is strengthened. In the case of preterm birth, however, 'doing everything possible' involves advising women to come in for assessment for every slight, possible symptom and recommending bed rest at home for those women whose symptoms are confirmed. Strengthening the legal position of the hospital may, therefore, shift a psychological, financial and personal burden on to women and their families, but this is rarely taken into consideration within the medical risk framework.

The triage record creates what is institutionally actionable and what is a 'private' responsibility. The condition of the woman's home situation or family resources falls outside the biomedical risk frame, and so social circumstances were not routinely assessed in triage or on the antepartum units. Yet poverty is well established as a determinant of health (Cooper 2002; Moss 2002; Van Kemenade 2003; Vissandjee et al. 2004; Walters 2004). It is also associated with premature labour and birth (Kramer et al. 2000; Pickett 1999). Despite what we know about the importance of poverty as a risk factor, poverty was rendered invisible in these institutional texts and work processes.

Deploying an individualised concept of biomedical risk in effect silenced women (Smith 1990). Women seldom volunteered information about financial and social resources unless asked directly. Of all the forms used in assessment and filled out with respect to women experiencing preterm labour, only one form gathered information about the social circumstances of the woman. This form was only filled out for women who were being admitted to the hospital; it had *one* question that asked about: 'family or friends nearby to help her once she is at home'. In contrast, the assessment of biomedical risk factors was included on *every* form and in the assessment of *every* woman. Furthermore, women were seldom asked about their occupation or work responsibilities in a way that entered this information into the clinical record. This omission may be related to the assumption that the woman at risk for preterm birth will quit work and 'stay home on bedrest' when she is told to do so.

Disciplining women

The identification of risk factors creates an opening for physicians and nurses to give medical advice to pregnant women. Nurses in triage were actively involved in teaching women diligence with self-surveillance and were observed to chastise women when their behaviours did not reflect the nurses' understandings of pregnancy risks.

A woman at 26 weeks gestation came into triage saying that she had slipped yesterday on the stairs and following this, had been leaking 'a lot' of clear fluid yesterday afternoon. Today, the leaking had stopped but her 'tail bone' was still sore. She shared with me that she had a three-year-old and 14 month old at home. She said that she did not know that she should have come in for assessment until she 'found her book' (*From Here Through Maternity*) later that evening. Leaking fluid was 'on the list' so she thought she should come in today to be checked 'just in case' (Triage Field notes 19 May 2004).

The nurse was very kind in her interactions with this woman, Connie. However, she also gave Connie some very clear messages that she *should* have come in yesterday for assessment. Afterwards, she explained to Karen that since this was Connie's third baby 'she ought to know better'. Apparently, Canadian women are expected to know about the 'risks' of leaking clear fluid. Connie is probably a very busy mother and may not have had the opportunity to reflect on her experience until the evening when her two young children were in bed. She would also have had to organise childcare for her two boys before she could come in to triage for assessment. None of this family 'context' information was entered on the triage record. Connie's everyday life experiences were rendered invisible and consequently irrelevant for her medical treatment.

The individualising discourses within the risk-ordered bio-medical framework resulted in nurses giving messages that implied judging or checking up on, rather than sharing responsibility with childbearing women. It is through these biomedical, institutional and nursing work processes that women are created as 'at risk' for preterm birth and are con-scripted into doing the work of keeping the baby in. This work includes continuing self-surveillance, suspending their lives when told to 'stop work and stay home on bed rest', and enlisting family support for their other care work responsibilities.

The effects of risk discourses on women's lives

Women in this study provided many instances where they picked up the message that preterm labour is caused by the woman's behaviour and bad lifestyle. The recruitment-into-surveillance literature provided by the health region emphasises that all pregnant women are at risk for preterm birth and so must monitor and promptly report symptoms. But in the same materials, the information on what women can do to reduce the risk of preterm birth highlights lifestyle 'choices' such as avoiding smoking, drinking, taking drugs, and so on. The four women in this study who gave birth early talked about the 'shame' of preterm birth, even those who had diligently avoided all the listed risk factors. For example, Eve couldn't understand why she had a preterm baby when she 'did everything right'. She provided examples of 'the kind of people they expect to be here [neonatal intensive care unit]' which included a prostitute who took drugs during pregnancy and a woman who didn't eat well because she was 'underpriv-ileged'. Eve said she felt ashamed for judging these women, but she was clearly drawing on local discourses about what 'you can do' to prevent preterm birth. 'What you *can* do' easily hardens into 'what you *should* do', thereby creating the category of 'those other mothers' who don't do a good job of caring for their developing babies. Khanya, a health professional whose first baby was born preterm, felt exposed and ashamed. She concluded that our culture sends a lot of messages that, if something goes wrong in pregnancy, it has to be 'the mom's fault'. Murphy (2000) noted that many preventive health strategies, such as the preterm birth prevention programme, are founded on assumptions of causal connections, responsibility and blame. There is an additional suffering in these women's accounts on top of the worry of having a preterm baby.

Despite coming from a variety of social locations and having different experiences with preterm labour, all the women in this study experienced suffering as a result of risk discourses. Vicki felt fear and guilt for doing too much or 'cheating' around prescribed bed rest. Lisa, on the other hand, felt guilty for *not* working. When Audrey was told to stay home on bed rest she felt punished and like she was 'in prison'. And Khanya felt 'judged' or stigmatised for having a preterm baby. Several women said that their assumptions of a normal pregnancy experience were disrupted by the preterm labour event; the pregnancy and their baby were now 'threatened' by their own bodies. These women's responses to 'going home on bed rest' included anxiety, fear and feeling alone with the responsibility. They talked about the work of 'keeping the baby in'. Sometimes this involved careful compliance with medical treatment including hospitalisation, decreased activity and bed rest. Some women were proactive and used strategies such as conscious relaxation and aromatherapy to help control their 'hostile' bodies. They also became much more conscious or aware of their body's signals. Overall, preterm labour was experienced by the women as a profound sense of personal responsibility for preventing preterm birth. Yet some of the women's financial and family circumstances made it difficult, if not impossible for them to 'be careful' in the ways the risk discourse promoted and that they felt themselves to be important.

For example, Vicki was the breadwinner for her family while her partner was in medical school. At the time of her interview, she was in her third pregnancy and had been hospitalised for preterm labour. She had also experienced preterm labour with her last pregnancy, and both her daughters had been born prematurely. Before she was discharged from the hospital this most recent time, she enquired whether homemaking assistance would be provided to help her care for her two pre-school children while maintaining bed rest.

> They were like ... and I asked about that and they just kind of looked at me like I was an alien and I thought, 'oh, just wondering.' Like I mean, like I don't know, it's just that I know there are times, and we're financially strapped because my husband is in school and stuff like that.

Vicki left the hospital without a referral for follow-up of any kind. Assessment of the woman's needs upon discharge was not part of the routine work process at the hospital. Referral for community follow-up was usually left to the discretion of the woman's doctor.

Vicki compared this experience of hospital discharge with the resources she had been offered when she experienced preterm labour four years ago in another Alberta city. That time she had received 30 hours each week of childcare assistance, along with nine hours of homemaking or housekeeping assistance. In contrast, the maximum amount of funded homemaking and childcare assistance available to her this time, if she was even referred to the regional antenatal home care program, was a total of nine hours per week. In Calgary, very limited assistance was available for women living with the threat of preterm labour, even women like Vicki who would, by any measure of biomedical risk, be considered 'high risk' for preterm birth.

Another woman's story highlighted the importance of financial resources and the legislative framework. Hope and her family were immigrants from Sudan and had lived in Canada for almost ten years. Her partner was a petroleum engineer, unemployed in his area of expertise, who had taken a less-skilled job to provide for his family. Hope held two part-time jobs. Their immediate family included their two-year-old daughter (born at term) and two teenage extended family members. At the time of her interview, Hope had recently given birth to a second daughter who was born very early. She had expected to work much longer during her pregnancy, as she had the first time. Now she was on government-funded maternity benefits, which amounted to 55 per cent of the income she had been earning before her maternity leave. Hers was the family's only income: her partner had been fired from his job when he missed three days of work during the time Hope was hospitalised with preterm labour and bleeding. Hope's family had exhausted their financial resources and simply could not make ends meet.

The provision of care for these women and families is grounded in assumptions that are made about women's lives based on a standardised model of the heterosexual family. Dorothy Smith (1999) describes the operations of this 'ideological code', which she calls SNAF or the Standard North American Family. SNAF assumes that every (decent) family has a male breadwinner/head of household and a wife-and-mother who, whether employed or not, makes family caregiving her priority. Smith describes how SNAF operates as a 'universalizing schema' and 'is not identifiable with any particular family; it applies to any' (Smith 1999: 159). SNAF-ordered discourses of preterm birth obscure the conflict between medical prescriptions of bed rest and some women's breadwinner responsibilities. Because in SNAF the woman's earnings are supplementary, early maternity leave is not presumed to cause financial hardship. But real women's ability to comply with bed rest treatment is directly linked to the financial resources of their families and the extent of the caregiving work their families require of them. That information about women's circumstances is not actively elicited with respect to treatment for preterm labour reveals the operation of SNAF, in a way that is detrimental to women in vulnerable situations.

Risk discourses intersect with economic and other social discourses that locate responsibility for caring work in the 'private' sphere. The assumption that the family is 'privately' responsible for care work in the home results in the lack of assessment of resources for managing the medical plan on discharge, and the lack of resources available or offered to assist families. Despite this gap in health care services, the responsibility for looking after small children in the home does not enter into the biomedical risk frame. Biomedical constructions of risk mask the disjuncture between the woman's everyday experiences and the possibilities for 'complying' with medical treatment plans that include the 'simple' treatment of 'staying home on bed rest'. The work of 'keeping the baby in' conflicts with family carework responsibilities and can cause significant hardships for some women and families. Perhaps hegemonic understandings of pregnancy as a 'choice' also limit women's entitlements to assistance during childbearing.

Discussion: what other understandings of pregnancy risks are possible?

This institutional ethnographic investigation has brought into view the organisation and the effects of multiple, interpenetrating discourses which together shape the everyday/everynight experiences of childbearing women and the nurses who work with them. The focus of the discussion has been on the way current discourses of risk and current practices of preterm birth prevention shift the burden of care to women and their families, in ways that can cause emotional suffering and financial hardship. There are two related issues here: how we understand risk in pregnancy and what level of support is made available to women experiencing preterm labour and preterm birth. Taking the standpoint of women suggests that addressing the problems identified in this study require attention to both.

Daviss (1997) developed a framework for analysing competing types of knowledge about childbirth that may be helpful for putting 'risk' discourses in their place. She states

> Technomedicine tends to look at decisions about birth in terms of levels of risk, rather than as decisions about choice of logic or about the conflicting claims to authority of different knowledge systems. Even when the medical system does acknowledge the existence of some of the categories, they are perceived as categories of risk – 'the clinical risk', 'the legal risk'. These are the authoritative categories in technomedicine, whereas cultural and personal factors are rarely acknowledged as being at risk. (Daviss 1997: 444)

Daviss proposed replacing the term 'risk' with the term 'logic': 'as an umbrella for our understanding of risk, benefit, and normalcy. To call these various priorities "types of logic" frames them in a non-threatening way and clarifies the need to recognize their competing claims to validity' (1997: 445). She also proposed multiple types of 'logic' scientific, clinical, personal, cultural, intuitive, political, legal and economic to help us think about pregnancy 'risks' in a more comprehensive way.

This study suggests that nurses and midwives need to be aware of the power of risk discourses over childbearing women so that they can begin to ease suffering and prevent 'spoiling' women's pregnancy and childbearing experiences with the *very loud discourses of risk*. Health care providers need to include the assessment of family resources and consider what assistance childbearing women might need to be successful in managing preterm labour *and* their caring work within their family. We need to provide women with an opportunity to talk about their family care work *and* occupational responsibilities *and* identify their concerns. We also need to include these women's stories in our accounts so that women's caring work becomes visible to the health care institution.

Conclusion

Making visible women's circumstances and documenting their need for support will, however, only be effective when there are additional social and economic resources in the community, so that women's actual needs can be matched with relevant assistance. Nurses and other health care providers can join with women in identifying and lobbying for needed policy change. For example, some women, such as university students, are currently not eligible for paid maternity benefits. Although pregnancy is a healthy state it is also a time when women are entitled to and need additional support. As well, nurses could be a strong voice in calling for more attention to the possible connection between employment conditions and preterm birth, and the establishment of legislation offering viable alternative work to pregnant women in strenuous jobs. Most importantly, as a society we need to change our thinking and discourses about risk and preterm birth prevention to include a sharing of responsibility. 'What *you* can do' needs to become 'What *we* can do' to prevent preterm birth.

7 Exploring the issues of risk and freedom for parents of children with life limiting, life threatening and chronic health problems

David Pontin

Introduction

The impetus for this chapter springs from my reflections and experiences of critical incidents in clinical practice, and may be seen as part of the movement for generating new nursing knowledge from lived experience (Rolfe 1998). As part of my work, I have links with a nursing service for children with life limiting (and life threatening) and chronic health problems (LLCHP). Over the past 15 years, the number of children surviving with LLCHP has increased. This is in part due to developments in health care technology and associated care practices, but also a shift in societal expectations and understandings of the issues faced by families (Emond and Eaton 2004). Consequently, more children with complex health care needs are being supported to live at home and to carry out the usual activities relevant to their peer group and cultural background (Kirk and Glendenning 2004; Lenton *et al.* 2001). Parents increasingly express their desire for their children to be cared for at home, and children living with these health challenges indicate that they want to be at home with their families and friends (Chambers and Oakhill 1995; Edwardson 1983; Martinson *et al.* 1986).

In the course of my work observing and talking with parents, children and colleagues, it struck me that many parents seemed to experience a tension in living with this situation. An important factor which seems to shape the way they care for their children is managing the possibly conflicting demands of the 'risks' to their children's health, while maintaining and providing a 'good' childhood. The tension seems to arise from the notion of a 'good' childhood, which includes the 'freedom' to explore and to experiment (Kelley *et al.* 1997), and parental (though usually mothers') concerns about maintaining a safe environment which would not compromise the health of their children (Van Dongen-Melman *et al.* 1998; Williams *et al.* 2003).

Connected to this seemed to be some of the issues faced by parents of children with disabilities, and the moral responsibility felt by parents, particularly mothers (McKeever and Miller 2004). The hegemony in contemporary western society is that children's well-being is determined by maternal action (Caplan 1998; Hays 1996). Mothering children with disabilities is sometimes pathologised for being overprotective and unrealistic, or mothers are accused of being in denial about the extent/impact of their children's condition (Ferguson 2001; Heiman 2002; Landsman 2003; Larson 1998; Phillip and Duckworth 1982; Read 2000) and it might be that beneath the surface this is the case for children with LLCHP. Work exploring parents' perspective on their care for their disabled children highlights that there is often a lack of appropriate social services/public services to support them (Darling 1979; Gliedman and Roth 1980; Phillip and Duckworth 1982). Kirk and Glendinning (2004) also suggest a similar picture for parents living with children with LLCHP, and it is this notion of risk that I want to explore further.

Late modernity

Chance and risk are the leitmotifs of late modern times, whose rationale is the control and subjugation of the natural world (Giddens 1990). The notion of risk is insidious and winds its way through social relations, influencing and shaping individual identity. In an attempt to ameliorate the consequences of external risk, various structural elements (social security, socialised healthcare systems, public housing) have been developed to minimise the effects of other's actions or uncontrollable forces. However, in late modernity, we know of risk in a particular form, as a form of risk that is manufactured through social action and organisation in post-industrial society with a shape-shifting character (Beck 1996).

In order for people to live with risk and make decisions about risk they need scientific or actuarial information on which to base their decisions and actions. The use of actuarial calculations is problematic because the probability of risk events, namely what we make happen, is mixed up with what happens (Giddens 1994). The assumption underlying risk society is that risk is everywhere and what we calculate is our degree of vulnerability. This raises some interesting questions when we consider the situations faced by parents of children with LLCHP. For example, what happens when the information that parents have confirms the fact that their children are unlikely to live into adulthood? Is there a telescoping effect whereby parents try to extend the limited time of their children's life available to them? Or are there other propositions open to them, such as do they make a conscious effort to promote a better quality of life with the risk of shortening the time available before the inevitable happens? In terms of the information that parents need, does having actuarial information make the decision making any easier or harder? In fact, do people use the actuarial information if it is available to them? There is an assumption in taking an actuarial position that the likelihood of specific health risks occurring can be aggregated to produce population risk figures which are then redistributed across individuals in a given population so that any benefits and burdens associated with the specific health risk are presumed to offset each other. An example that helps to illustrate this is immunisation. For each immunisation event there is a risk of adverse consequences for individuals, but the benefits and burdens of adverse risks are thought to compensate for each other, the risk of vaccine damage to a minority is worth the risk to prevent major infectious disease epidemics. However, at the individual level this view is misleading because health outcomes cannot be distributed across individuals; if I am going to die or be damaged by a vaccine, then only I shall die or be damaged, none else shares that outcome. Therefore, it would seem that the risks seen by individuals are understated in any population-based, actuarial model (Asch and Hershey 1995).

Concerns about safety run deep through the core of risk society and this manifests itself as anxiety in people because problems are invisible until the detrimental consequences spring forth (Beck 1992). There is a complicated dialectical relationship with science in risk society. At one and the same time, science can both feed and assuage anxieties. There is a paradox in that it has the potential to identify risk factors, exacerbate risky situations by scientific advances and developments, and also produce ways in which risks may be ameliorated and reduced. This paradox of science could be seen to be experienced in a number of ways by parents and children living with LLCHP. First, there are the differing opinions that may be sought or given by a variety of medical practitioners as families search for diagnoses that reflect their concerns. Second, there is the dilemma of using newly conceived interventions or treatments when they are still in their beta-testing phase. Finally, there is the use of palliative care skills that allow children to live into death. Having looked at the notion of risk, I now move on to some of the implications for welfare structures and professional working practices.

Risk, late modernity and welfare structures

Although the restructuring process of late modernity has been fraught and problematic, throughout advanced industrial capitalist societies, the Fordist factory structures which were characteristic of early modern industrial capitalism, have changed to a post-Fordist organisation of production. These changes have been replicated in the structure, form and orientation of welfare systems and the way risk in the lives of vulnerable or dangerous individuals is managed (Hirsch 1991; Tomaney 1994). The institutional structures of early modernity, which segregated the general population from the recipients of services, have been replaced with service delivery systems that do not necessarily have coherent, boundaried, physical structures.

Instead, networks, frameworks and pathways have been constructed to provide 'care in the community' (Alaszewski *et al.* 1997; Swift and Pontin 2001). An example of this can be seen in the deinstitutionalisation and normalisation of managing care arrangements for children with LLCHP made over the last 20 years (Chambers and Oakhill 1995; Edwardson 1983; Emond and Eaton 2004; Lenton *et al.* 2001; Martinson *et al.* 1986) and the development of managed clinical networks (Kunkler 2000).

The structural changes in welfare provision have had a particular effect on the management processes of risk. There is an increasing focus on client welfare, and in particular on child care. It seems wholly ironic that, while authors such as Furedi (2001) berate parents for their concerns about safety and managing risk for the welfare of their children, the act of berating parents in itself may be seen as part of the late modern project with the emphasis on individuation, personal responsibility and challenging the traditional authority of health professionals. These processes which characterise the late modern condition (Beck 1992) may be seen in the contradictory relationship that co-exists between the extent of risk and what is available to professionals for its management. As the extent of the risk to which clients are exposed increases, the means for actually resolving the situation become less certain. There is a societal expectation that professionals should clearly identify the nature of risk that clients may encounter and then to manage the risk even though their professional authority to take appropriate actions may be unclear (Alaszewski *et al.* 1997).

The rationale for maintaining individuals in usual, although riskier, community settings but with professionals still responsible for managing the risk elements, takes us straight to the heart of the late modern project – the notions of individualism, normalisation, and civil rights (Department of Health (DoH) 1989). Such situations may be seen in the care of children who are technology dependent. There are children who, ten years ago would, at worst, not be alive or at best, be living in high dependency/ intensive care units on a long-term basis, who are now cared for at home by their parents, family members, carers and nurses. Even though they are living at home and parents are encouraged to 'normalise' the surroundings and make things as usual as possible, the professionals still retain the responsibility for managing the risk, for example, technology failure (Kirk and Glendenning 2004).

A major risk management dilemma that professionals have to address is the reality that trying to gauge levels of risk is not a straightforward, unproblematic, technical activity. It is difficult to formulate objective risk measures when the phenomena are categorised as low probability-high consequence, lightning striking an individual twice (Douglas 1992). Professionals in these situations find themselves in a classic double bind scenario. They are subject to public criticism if they 'over protect' individuals and yet, they are scapegoated if the client or public are harmed in anyway. There are times when the notion of over protection may be construed as a rational and logical response by parents to a low probability but high consequence category. Such a situation might arise when a child is immuno-compromised and parents choose not to immunise against childhood illnesses as the vaccine may pose a greater risk than the possibility of exposure to 'wild' virus (Royal College of Paediatrics & Child Health 2002). The key tipping point of community care is based on finding and supporting a reasonable balance between promoting and enhancing individual freedom and providing protection (Brearley 1982; Swift and Pontin 2001). From my observations and reflections on practice, and conversations with clinical colleagues and parents, it would seem that this is the point at issue for parents of children with LLCHP. There is a need and desire to promote the circumstances for children to explore life and the world around them, whilst making sure that the roots of security and stability are present for their children to experience a 'good' childhood and at the same time being mindful of the possible implications for their health and longevity.

It may be that parents find themselves in a situation where they want, and need to encourage the development of individual freedom in their children. In this way, the individuals concerned have the opportunity to develop their potential to the maximum in the short time they have, and to enjoy their life. However, at the same time, the very activities that contribute to making fulfilling and satisfactory experiences may hasten the demise of individual children. By encouraging and facilitating increased autonomy in children living with LLCHP, parents and professionals charged with managing the risk find themselves in the paradox where there is a corresponding increase in risk which cannot be prevented. Beck makes the point that risk society members learn to manage the anxiety inherent in their situation (Beck 1992). What is not clear from the literature on families living with children facing LLCHP is: how do they learn to manage the anxiety of a more manifest situation? Their children are going to die – it is just a question of when and how? If the process of individuation in risk society highlights individual responsibility to control the factors, how do parents of children with LLCHP go about this? To what extent are their actions driven by the notion that parents are morally responsible for their children's development (McKeever and Miller 2004)? One way in which people are said to manage the situation of late modernity is by risk assessment (Beck 1992), I now want to move on to explore whether people's perception of risk leads to the manufacture of hazards.

Do risk perceptions manufacture hazards?

Fox (1998) maintains that hazards are created by people, and that hazards originate from their situation-specific judgements about outcomes that may be inauspicious for them. In this respect, hazards are used to estimate risk, weigh up risky behaviour and to make judgements about people who take risks. According to this argument, the materialisation of hazards happens once some forms of adverse events are identified.

This constructionist account maintains that hazards are brought into existence by the conscious act of analysing risks (Wells 1996). Concessions are made that the events and objects may be real, but in and of themselves, the events and objects are not hazards. They become hazardous only in circumstances where their qualities are perceived by people to have a detrimental effect on themselves or others, objects or the events surrounding them. These judgements are based on this change from inert status to being hazardous and the change happens as a result of our judgement that an adverse situation may arise from exposure to the object or events. An example that may illustrate this point that has come to the forefront in many schools in the United Kingdom (UK) is the presence of peanuts or nuts in school environs. Peanuts and nuts are inert items; they become hazardous only when a person who exhibits an anaphylactic or anaphylactoid response comes into physical contact with them or a product which contains traces of them. Therefore the act of risk assessment, namely finding out if anyone exhibits gross immunological responses to peanuts or nuts, brings them into the category of hazard.

People's judgement about hazard and risk may be based on their personal or vicarious experience, or an authoritative body of knowledge (discourse) namely risk assessment. If the risk assessment indicates a very low probability of the hazard happening, then the inert object or event is not construed as a hazard. So if there are no children in the school with a nut or peanut allergy, then there is no hazard. Of course, this raises the question of how do you know that you are or are not allergic if you've never been exposed? This process of judging probability is incremental. It depends on prior judgements having been made about hazards, otherwise it becomes an impossible task with everything labelled as hazardous because everything has a risk potential. Such a situation is shown when the consequences of risk have to be addressed which previously were not identified (Suter 1993).

This is a situation that parents of children living with LLCHP face. Previously innocuous situations become the subject of assessment about whether they are hazardous or not and parents have to work out the risk to their children. This raises questions about whether parents develop prioritisation systems to analyse the risk presented to their children so that they do not become overwhelmed by the risk assessment task? If so, is this a conscious activity and how do they go about establishing the parameters? What type of information is used – scientific (establishment or peripheral), actuarial, vicarious? If it is not an explicit conscious activity, how do they respond to the challenges that everyday life throws up? Are there health sequelae for parents in managing risk probabilities? And are these gendered as one might suspect with mothers experiences being different from fathers (Shore *et al.* 2004)?

There is also an assumption that risk assessment is a one off process – the school has been assessed and it has no children on the books with nut allergy, therefore there is no or very low hazard. But of course, the school population ebbs and flows and has termly tidal eddies. Children move out of the area, move into the area, new cohorts start each autumn and also leave. In some respects we might expect the risk assessment process to be continuous at a low level or at least a series of discrete events, but is this the case? There is also an assumption that the children affected are themselves in a static situation, but by their very nature of being children, they are in a state of becoming. What is a high risk at one age may be less of a risk at another as bodies grow, cognition alters and understanding about the world deepens. It is unreasonable to assume that nursery class children can take effective avoidance action to limit contact with nut products in the same way as seven-year-old children can. We expect the latter to be able to tell us clearly about their situation and take some self-preservative avoidance action. This gives us some imagined indication of the shape-shifting aspect of the manufactured risks prevalent for children, but a closer examination of how risk is assessed and hazards materialised in children's homes and their schools, would allow us to explore the ways in which parents manage the anxiety of living in risky situations.

It may be that risk assessment for parents starts with what is usually in the realm of the probable in every day life but infused with new knowledge or sets of assumptions based on their new or revised situation of living with LLCHP. The source of this knowledge may be their own experience from recent or distant times; vicarious experience gained directly from others or mediated by discussion boards on the internet; scientific sources or professional sources which may be either hegemonic or challenging. Either way, it seems that the decisions parents have to make are contextual and conditional to time and place (Wynne 1992). A major issue that may be worthy of investigation here is whether there is a divergence between parents and others over what is acknowledged as a risk and a hazard. Are there different knowledge positions that prevent agreement on what constitutes evidence to confirm or disconfirm hazardous situations? Does this alter depending on the issue which affects the children? One strand of inquiry here is making sense of parental behaviour and in the next section I want to explore health lifestyles and understanding parental behaviour.

Health lifestyles and understanding parental behaviour

If it is anything, then risk society may be seen as people living with a sense of risk that affects all aspects of their everyday lives (Beck 1996). This is echoed and reflected in health promotion perspectives which acknowledge that any aspect of everyday life poses risks to health of a greater or lesser extent but certain human activities have more far ranging effects than others, for example, smoking, unprotected penetrative sex (Nettleton 1997; Petersen 1997). Health lifestyles may be conceptualised as a complex interaction that takes place between the life chances and life choices which are available to people as a condition of their socio-economic resources (Cockerham *et al.* 1997). Woven through these interactions between life chances and life choices are the notions of self-control and moral worth signified by one's behaviour (Harding 1997). Bourdieu's notions of habitus, field, position and capital have been used by McKeever and Miller (2004) and Shore *et al.* (2004) to explore the mothering of children with chronic health problems. McKeever and Miller use the concepts of habitus, field and capital to explore maternal behaviour as a form of social reproduction and struggle to resist devalued bodily capital (Wacquant 1995). However, this resistance may also be viewed as a form of risk strategy to avoid stigma (Green 2003). McKeever and Miller suggest that mothers' actions are logical strategies that include and reject the devalued social positioning of disabled children. Their strategies include acquiescing at times to dominant players in the field of children's medicine and long-term care, managing children's presentation and positioning in social space, and enhancing children's bodily posture and carriage.

Habitus may be thought of as our understandings of life which form the backdrop to the main action. This explains how individuals develop knowledge of expectations about behaviour in different social settings, and thinking and feeling in different aspects of everyday life. People change their behaviour and objectives according to their understanding and expectation of anticipated consequences, namely life chances pertinent to their social position (Bourdieu and Wacquant 1992). With regard to parents of children with LLCHP, we would expect there to be changes to their habitus as a consequence of their children's shortened life expectancy. The notion of habitus allows us to develop a sense of one's place and a sense of the place of others relative to oneself in different social situations (Bourdieu 1995). It may be thought of as a scheme to reproduce and generate individual expression within social order as well as generating and reproducing the social order itself (Bourdieu and Wacquant 1992). It may be at this juncture that parents feel the tension between risk and freedom. Depending on the changes to their habitus, they may experience the strength to create a 'good' childhood for their children, or conversely experience structural constraints and conform to expected norms.

This view of social action can be criticised for being deterministic and denying the possibility that social order may be altered by structural action, addressing social inequities and poverty (James 2000; Prout 2000). However, it has been suggested that habitus is not a deterministic mechanism, and that it can bring about improvisation, and resistance to hegemony (Lahire 2003; Marcoulatos 2001; Meisenhelder 1997; Swartz 1997). While people's lives are shaped and directed to a greater or lesser degree by social structures and historical forces, people have the capacity for individual and social transformation by the use of various forms of capital. This may be seen in McKeever and Miller's work where mothers managed the social positioning of their children by managing their presentation through posture and bodily carriage.

In the Bourdieusian sense, capital may be seen as resources, goods and values which are available to people in different positions in different fields. There are four generic types – economic (inherited or generated wealth), cultural (educational qualifications, aesthetic preferences, bodily characteristics, speech/dialect), social (networks, group memberships) and symbolic (role, legitimacy, authority and prestige). The types of capital which are available for people to use may be material or symbolic, and the value of the capital is set by the logic and characteristics of specific fields at particular times (Bourdieu 1990). The use of capital may be seen in Shore *et al.* (2004) and their work with families whose children lived with epilepsy. Mothers of children with chronic epilepsy appear to adapt positively. This is despite the fact that they, worry about long-term sequelae of the condition and its treatment (Austin *et al.* 1995), and there is the possibility of over-protection and social isolation due to stigma (Carlton-Ford *et al.* 1997; Eiser *et al.* 1992). Mothers learn the rules of the game to the extent that they are confident in managing seizures so that they can take risks in managing children's conditions to maintain usual family life.

Field refers to the social and symbolic institutions (such as family, medicine, law and education) that make up social life. The positions people occupy in different fields depend on the relative power of their habitus within the field. When people are located within a particular field they carry out expected game-like behaviour that reproduces or changes the transformation of power/resources in a particular field. To be socially adept and successful, players must learn the rules of the game that form the logic for the attitudes and behaviour for a given field. It may be that some parents are able to learn a greater repertoire of rules about being parents of children with LLCHP because of the range of capital at their disposal. This might be an instance where the creative improvisation of the habitus comes to the fore.

Another way of examining the relationship between lifestyle, life chance and life choice is by using the notion of arche-health (Fox 1998). Arche-health may be conceived of as a process that emphasises the transformative nature of human life and experience and rejects the idea of a single identity being attributed to a thing or a person. It works on the premise that people have a dynamic nature and are not fixed. Instead of talking about human beings, arche-health refers to human becoming and may be complementary with

Parse's (1987) theory of nursing. Because transformation allows variation to flourish, arche-health suggests that phenomena which might previously have been perceived as fixed move into flux and that a variety of meanings around health/illness may be generated. Arche-health can be seen in people's behaviour in a number of ways, such as when they act and choose to behave in ways to normalise bodily functions. An example here is Green's work on living with cerebral palsy (Green 2003). Alternatively, it offers carers the opportunities to support people in enacting the choices which promote human becoming which may be obstructed by illness or disability (Fox 1995).

The choice that is referred to here draws on the notion of an individualistic, rational actor but it also acknowledges that choices may be unpredictable, unwitting, or united with others. At one and the same time, choice in this context has the possibility of being an act of defiance and denial and a positive declaration; all of these are processes of human becoming, namely arche-health. If we use the notion of arche-health to gaze at the situation faced by parents of children with LLCHP, then it is possible to see risk and health as part of a late modern discourse which has the potential for people to resist constraining cultural constructions on how dying children should be parented. Risk taking by some parents and children may be seen as the active process of choosing as life unfolds. For parents of children with LLCHP the unfolding is very real. It may be short and intense with each risk having a dramatic twist in the tale/ but it is the embodiment of human becoming.

Conclusion

This chapter has drawn on my experiences of working with families and children living with LLCHP and explored the notion of risk and freedom. That exploration of risk has centred on the need and desire of parents to promote the circumstances for their children to explore life and the world around them, whilst making sure that the roots of security and stability are present for their children to experience a 'good' childhood and at the same time being mindful of the possible implications for their health and longevity. Along the way, I have explored the avenues for further formal inquiry, as well as located this project within a wider discourse by juxtaposing ideas of risk from Beck and Giddens with concepts drawn from Bourdieu and Fox. There appears to be a number of strands of inquiry that might be productive for nursing practice, in particular exploring parents' use of information when choosing how to parent children whose lifespan may be short.

8 The tension between autonomy and safety in nursing adults with learning disabilities

Bob Heyman and
Jacqueline Davies

Introduction

This chapter will discuss the role of the nurse in risk management for adults with learning disabilities, drawing on research undertaken by the first author in a variety of care and treatment contexts over the last decade. A social science approach to risk, as outlined by Godin in Chapter 1, will be adopted. This approach views a risk framework as a culturally mediated but variable perspective which social actors, including adults with learning disabilities, their friends and relatives and professional carers, may draw upon in order to understand their condition and attempt to manage their future. Nursing per se will not be the principal focus of the chapter. Learning disability nursing is a recognised sub-profession (Coyle and Northway 1999; Shirtliffe 1995), although the number of specialist learning disability nurses has declined substantially, in the United Kingdom (UK) at least, since publication of the Jay Report (Jay 1979). Nurses work with adults with learning disabilities in diverse specialist and generic contexts, as outlined below. Mostly, they operate in a multidisciplinary context, particularly since large residential institutions have been closed down in the UK and elsewhere. It is hoped that, despite this relative dearth of specific reference, nurses will find the chapter useful in terms of developing a critical understanding of issues associated with nursing care.

In the inevitably sketchy and illustrative discussion which follows, we will first raise the issue of the construction of adults with learning disabilities as risk entities; outline the current living circumstances of adults with learning disabilities; and then consider the dilemma of autonomy *versus* safety, which is central to risk management in all contexts.

Constructing people with learning disabilities as a risk entity

Before the risks faced and posed by adults with learning disabilities can be identified, assessed and managed, the category of people must be recognised as a risk entity. This point may seem laboured and obvious. However, risk entities are given that status by cultural groups who recognise them as such. In doing so, members of a society perform a number of implicit operations which, because they are taken-for-granted and implicit, shape subsequent responses. Constructing a risk entity entails differentiation, marking out a category as distinctive, homogenisation, treating members of the category as similar, and valorisation, attaching value to the constructed entity. This act of classification applies to sub-categories of adults with learning disabilities, since the term covers a vast range, from people with severe and profound disabilities who have little or no linguistic capacity through to those whose cognitive impairment is marginal, and whose status as learning-disabled is heavily influenced by the circumstances of their upbringing. Anyone who works or shares their life with an adult with a learning disability or any other labelled condition recognises their individuality. Nevertheless, categorisation does mark out particular groups who, in early twenty-first century risk-obsessed societies, are viewed in terms of a presumed risk profile.

The politics of classification, and the implicit value judgements which underpin this action, can be traced through terminological variation. In the UK, in general, health professionals, including nurses working in the National Health Service (NHS), use the term learning disability, whilst social services prefer the term learning difficulties. Historically, these terms have, in the UK at least, replaced labels such as 'mentally disordered' and 'mentally subnormal' which have become stigmatised. Eayrs *et al.* (1993) found that 'people with learning difficulties' were viewed more favourably than 'the mentally handicapped' or the 'mentally subnormal'. The former were also viewed as less in need of special provision, a paradoxical consequence of reduced stigmatisation.

The currently used terms are nuanced differently, since the term learning disability locates presumed problems within the individual to a greater extent than the term learning difficulty, since a difficulty can arise from the person, the environment or their interaction. For example, a person may experience a learning difficulty because they are badly taught. Crucially, assumptions, often tacit and unarticulated, about the extent to which health and welfare issues are located in an individual classified as having a disability, as against the environment in which they live, will shape the ways in which others, including health services, respond to these issues. The idea of a disabling society (Oliver 1990) neatly reverses the implicit assumption that the 'problem' is located in the person with a disability. For example, if people with learning disabilities are offered similar time with a GP to that allotted to those who can communicate more quickly, the access of the former to health care will inevitably suffer. The nature of solutions to this problem will depend upon whether it is initially viewed as resulting from the failure of the health care system to allocate additional resources, which would enable health care professionals to spend more time with individual patients, or the failure of some people with learning disabilities to communicate at the required pace. These are not necessarily exclusive alternatives, and the former is not self-evidently preferable, since allocating more of a scarce resource such as GP, or nursing, time to one group must inevitably take it away from others. The example does illustrate the dangerous implications of prior assumptions which can inhibit imaginative consideration of alternative options. The term 'learning disabilities' will be used in this chapter simply because of its wide acceptance by UK health professionals and its closeness to the internationally used label of 'intellectual disabilities'.

Given these caveats, adults with learning disabilities as a socially defined category of people, can be seen as subject to a wide range of health-related risks, which include:

Being subject to abuse (Baker and Allen 2001)
Being physically unfit (Messent *et al.* 1999)
Having a poor quality diet (Bryan *et al.* 2000)
Socially isolated (Chappell 1994)
Experiencing mental health problems (Morgan 2003)
Experiencing physical health problems (Kerr *et al.* 1996).

As the entire population is liable to experience adverse events of these sorts, asserting that people with learning disabilities are 'at risk' entails proposing that people with learning disabilities face an unacceptably higher than normal probability of experiencing them. Such propositions require a definition of what constitutes an unacceptable level of risk, a contentious issue, as will be illustrated below. Moreover, such risk propositions are based on observations or beliefs about populations, but are applied to individuals. Stereotyping and mismatches between risk categorisation and the capabilities of individuals often result from this mode of thought. For example, although adults with learning disabilities are at greater risk of social isolation, some have supportive social networks (Mest 1988).

Life and care contexts

Adults with learning disabilities live in a variety of settings, hospitals, care homes, supported housing and their own home or that of their parents. They may be married, have children and work with varying degrees of protection. Some attend day centres, but, in the UK and no doubt elsewhere, this form of provision for people with disabilities has been reduced over the last two decades (Department of Health (DoH) 2000c). For adults with learning disabilities, day centre activities, often ill-matched to individual aspirations (Whittaker and McIntosh 2000), have been replaced by care packages which encourage, in theory at least, greater integration with the wider community. Similarly, large residential hospitals have been almost entirely closed down, being used only for those with very special needs, for example, serious offenders with learning disabilities for whom medium secure health services provide an alternative to prison. The new value placed on people with learning disabilities taking risks is associated with prevailing ideas about normalisation (Wolfensberger 1972), although it should not be assumed that a more sheltered life is necessarily safer or better.

More generally, over the last 20 years, people with learning disabilities have come to be viewed, at the level of policy statements, at least (Manthorpe 2001), as citizens with human rights, the exercise of which entails the acceptance of risks, rather than as dependent, vulnerable people in need of protection. Nurses and other professional carers are expected to embrace choice and risk taking for this client group (Sines 1995, Parrish and Styring 2003). However, as will be argued below, the new culture of risk taking is not always welcomed by adults with learning disabilities and family carers. Professional carer missionary zeal in favour of risk taking needs to be tempered by sympathetic appreciation of the perspectives of those whom professionals seek to 'liberate', not necessarily in accordance with their clients' wishes, from a more protective culture.

Hospital residents, often with severe and profound learning disabilities, have been decanted into smaller 'community' facilities located in urban areas. However, the community label should not be confused with true social integration which may or may not take place in different life zones. Community facilities have been characterised as '*archipelagos of care*', isolated pockets of institutionalisation. For example, carers in community facilities for adults with severe learning disabilities were observed to adopt a precautionary approach to risk management based on the problems posed by the most risky individual (Corkish and Heyman 1998). The door of one community home was locked because one resident was prone to run out onto the busy road fronting the home. In this case, a flexible solution was found, an electronic locking system which could only be operated by the more able residents. In another home, the kitchen had been locked because one resident had nearly choked after attempting to eat a loaf of bread with its wrapper still on.

Such precautionary risk management strategies may be necessitated by the requirement to care for groups of vulnerable adults *en masse*. Nevertheless, they give rise to some ironic contrasts with phased-out care in large, rural residential hospitals where adults with severe learning disabilities can roam free from traffic risks, although they may face other hazards there, such as being sexually abused or exploited. More generally, the use of high-tech resources such as satellite tracking devices may be seen as a means of reconciling safety with autonomy for people with learning disabilities and other potential members of vulnerable groups. However, their use needs to be carefully considered in relation to issues of human rights and dignity (Welsh *et al.* 2003).

Even when not physically separated from the wider community, adults with learning disabilities are more likely than the rest of the population to experience poor integration with respect to employment (Jenkins 2002), social relationships (Chappell 1994) and access to health services (Coyle and Northway 1999). Social isolation is perhaps the biggest risk faced by adults with learning disabilities who may be ignored by non-disabled peers and unable to maintain relationships even with peers with learning disabilities because of transport and other mobility restrictions. Attempts to cope with the damaging psychosocial consequences of social isolation, for example, through the generation of fantasy relationships or adoption of a short-term fatalistic attitude to life may be dismissed as symptomatic of a learning disability, with the consequence that serious mental health problems are not detected (Heyman *et al.* 1997).

Although health services are free and supposedly universal in the UK, adults with learning disabilities experience poorer access to health care than the rest of the population, despite being at greater risk of health problems, as noted above. Ensuring that adults with learning disabilities receive equitable access to health services requires inclusion rather than mere integration. For example, if GPs and other primary care professionals offer equal time to all patients regardless of their communication skills, adults with learning disabilities who need more time to express themselves will lose out. Our qualitative research (Heyman *et al.* 2004) identified subtle exclusionary processes. For example, one respondent, recently relocated from a residential hospital to a community residence, visited the optician without an appointment, and was told that she would need to return on another occasion. Community members with a better understanding of the working of health services would have asked for an appointment. More tellingly, they would not have left the optician without being offered one. This woman had not got round to revisiting the optician and had, in effect, been discouraged from using a service to which she was entitled. Access to health care in residential settings may be no less problematic (Goodman *et al.* 2003), but depends upon organisational factors rather than the capabilities of individuals.

The risks which adults with learning disabilities see themselves (or are seen as) facing vary widely, depends upon their capabilities and living circumstances. The section which follows will explore risk management generically, drawing upon the idea that risk management entails balancing autonomy with safety.

The dilemma of autonomy versus safety

Given that people with learning disabilities are constituted as a risk entity, and seen as being at higher risk of experiencing adverse events such as those outlined above, health and social care systems may be seen as having a role to play in managing such risks, reducing their prevalence closer to acceptable levels. Risk management can be usefully understood in terms of dealing with the dilemma of autonomy versus safety (Baldwin and Thirkettle 1999). This dilemma, conceived at the broadest possible level, arises when risk management, formal or informal, limits personal freedom in an attempt to avoid or reduce risks judged to be unacceptable. The autonomy *versus* safety dilemma comes into play when increasing safety levels reduces autonomy levels and vice versa. For example, pregnant women might be offered home delivery, conventional hospital care or high intensity surveillance. High surveillance might be seen as safest, but also as offering women the smallest degree of control over the delivery of their baby. Such analyses tend to be highly controversial. For instance, the extra safety offered by hospital over home deliveries has been questioned (Tew 1990) in relation to the potential iatrogenic (health-damaging) impact of the former.

However, the general point to be made is that people with learning disabilities, family carers and human service organisations manage risk by offering different balances between safety and autonomy. All of the above are risk managers in the sense that they think about and attempt to deal with risks, not only to the adult with learning disabilities, but also to themselves and others. For example, health and social care professionals may be concerned about career damage and litigation. The theory of risk management insists that properly assessed risks are acceptable but in practice serious adverse events tend to trigger enquiries which apportion blame with the benefit of hindsight which was not available to the risk taker. Family carers, who professionals encourage to accept that their son or daughter should take risks, may feel that the consequences of managing any adverse consequences will fall on them, not the professionals. According to the cultural theory of risk (Douglas 1966), the dangers which a culture chooses to worry about reflect its underlying values. Within a particular cultural context, risk selection is influenced by personal interest and orientation.

Risk managers, in the broad sense defined above, tend to assume that a more restricted and regulated environment is less risky, locating life settings within a particular domain in a hierarchy of risk. For example, living at home might be considered less risky than living in sheltered accommodation which, in turn, is judged safer than living independently. Such judgements are not necessarily objectively correct. For instance, an adult with learning disabilities living in sheltered accommodation might be subject to abuse from staff. Someone who is living in the parental home against his wishes might experience depression. The outcome of risk assessment depends upon what risks are selected for consideration, as noted above. All too often, the assumptions on which risk management is predicated are not themselves reflected upon, leaving the outcome dependent on assumptions which might not stand up to critical analysis.

Four important issues associated with attempted balancing of safety with autonomy will be noted. First, identifying the optimum balance between safety and autonomy for an individual depends upon risk assessment which may be formal and/or informal. As the assessed riskiness of the person increases, so the presumed optimal balance between safety and autonomy will shift towards safety. However, judgements about riskiness need to take on board wider personal characteristics and the qualitative features of cognitive impairment, as illustrated by the quotation below.

> *Family carer:* The educational part of her brain is alright, but the social side is damaged. (Heyman and Huckle 1993b: 155)

Family carers may emphasise such qualitative differences to a greater extent than health and social care professionals because of their greater personal experience with the individual who is being risk managed. As noted above, risk analysis tends to homogenise members of a constructed category. Professionals may tend to think about risk in more generic terms, as illustrated by the following quotation.

> *Paid carer (day centre):* We are all subject to risk, and they will not learn without taking risk. (Heyman and Huckle 1993a: 1562)

Second, risk managers assess risks in a broader context of informal, intuitive cost benefit analysis. The acceptability of a risk is judged in terms of its anticipated benefits as well as the probability of something going wrong. For example, some of the family carers who participated in our study and who considered independent travel too risky for the adult with learning disabilities whom they cared for, also maintained that this form of autonomy was not really needed.

> *Family carer:* I think she comes home from work tired and, in our terms, she's a bit overweight. She is glad of a sit down when she comes in. She doesn't want to go out and do anything physical any more. (Heyman and Huckle 1995: 175)

By devaluing the benefits of autonomy, family carers could lessen the perceived cost of opting for safety. However, adults with learning disabilities will not necessarily make the same judgement since the impact of this risk management strategy falls most directly on them. This type of difference in perspective is illustrated by the next quotation, from the daughter of the respondent quoted above.

> *Adult with learning disabilities:* Yes, I would like to see [friends], but I don't have a chance to see [friend]. (Heyman and Huckle 1995: 176)

As documented in the last example, an important consideration in any cost benefit analysis is the anticipated direction of adverse consequences. Risks affect those involved with their management in different ways. In general, risk managers, in the broad sense defined above, may feel more ready to accept risks which do not impact directly on their own lives. The day centre staff interviewed for the research referenced above recommended risk taking in zones outside their own remit, for example, travelling, working or living independently. The attitudes of family carers vary substantially. However, they may be resistant to accepting risks pressed upon them by professional carers.

> *Family carer:* Every time I go to the [clinical] review [meeting], they keep saying it is time she got a job. But she is epileptic, and could not work in a kitchen. I tell them what she is like. I should know. I made her. (Heyman and Huckle 1993a: 1562)

Some family carers pointed out that they, not care professionals, would have to deal with the consequences if risk taking led to adverse consequences. The parent quoted below feared that her son would be left with nothing if he accepted the risk of taking a job which did not work out.

> *Family carer:* I wouldn't want him to get a job and then find out he didn't like it, because then he couldn't get his place back at the [day] centre straight away. It took us a year to get [adult] a place in here in the first place. (Heyman and Huckle 1995: 180)

Nurses and other professional carers need to appreciate the perspectives of those who live with a sense of pervading risk arising from the perceived vulnerability of their son or daughter. Paid carers may be markedly less risk-tolerant when risks of litigation, for example, affect them directly.

A third issue related to safety/autonomy balances is that the terms of their tradeoff are not fixed. Skilful interventions can reduce the level of risk associated with a given level of autonomy, or increase the amount of autonomy which can be achieved at a given level of risk. If people with learning disabilities are seen as vulnerable in certain situations, then the situations can be made safer or an individual's skills can be enhanced, so that he or she becomes better able to manage risks.

One way in which the risks associated with a given level of autonomy can be reduced is by differentiating situations, so that the most risky are ruled out. For example, parent participants in our study who allowed their adult son or daughter to go out on their own often differentiated safer and less safe environments, excluding the latter.

> *Family carer:* I wouldn't want him to go night-clubbing.
>
> *Interviewer:* Why is that?
>
> *Family carer:* I don't know, but I just prefer him to be at the pub. I'd rather him be among the people he knows. (Heyman *et al.* 1998: 208)

In contrast, parents and other family carers who judged a risk unacceptable tended to generalise its dangerousness, sometimes drawing on single instances as evidence, as illustrated in the next quotation.

> *Family carer:* It's this element of being protective really, because once upon a time there was a case in [local town] where this little girl had got on the bus, and she did not know that she had not got off the bus until she reached [town about 30 miles away]. She had gone to sleep on the back seat. It's that type of thing. As much as you would like her to use it [public transport independently], I don't know if it is worth the hassle. (Heyman *et al.* 1998: 208)

This respondent had generalised from an incident involving a child to the circumstances of her adult daughter. In general, multiple conclusions, supporting different risk management decisions, can be reasonably drawn from the same 'evidence'. Health and social care professionals need to take account of the frameworks of risk understanding utilised by clients and carers. The quoted respondent might have modified her cost benefit analysis for the risk of her daughter travelling independently, if she had been helped to differentiate situations in which this form of autonomy would be more or less risky.

Fourth, and finally, management of the safety *versus* autonomy dilemma needs to be understood in its interpersonal micro-political context. The latter term is used because, as already illustrated in relation to disputes between family carers and day centre staff, divergences of views about risk management tend to be highly charged. We classified 20 families in terms of the attitude of the main family carer (usually a parent) and the adult with learning disabilities towards risks affecting the latter (Heyman and Huckle 1995).

In 11 families, both parties were classified as risk-averse, agreeing, for example, that it was too dangerous for the adult with learning disabilities to travel or live independently, as illustrated by the following pair of quotations from interviews undertaken independently with an adult with learning disabilities and his mother.

> *Interviewer:* Would you like to be able to go out on your own?
>
> *Adult with learning disabilities:* No.
>
> *Interviewer:* Why?
>
> *Adult with learning disabilities:* It's very dangerous.
>
> *Interviewer:* Can [son] use public transport on his own?
>
> *Mother:* No. I have never allowed him to travel on a bus on his own. I would worry too much. It's a difficult situation. (Heyman *et al.* 1998: 205)

As illustrated by the second quotation, family carers bring their own very real feelings of anxiety into their cost-benefit calculations, so that worry about risks becomes a factor influencing decision making.

Family carers who leaned towards safety were sometimes concerned not only with the direct risks associated with particular forms of autonomy, but also with new areas of risk which they might give rise to.

> *Mother:* I don't like him doing too much, you know. If he can [travel to work independently], maybe the next thing, he can start and go up [elsewhere] by himself. (Heyman *et al.* 1998: 207)

Eleven families were characterised as risk acceptors who took on certain risks despite concerns about adverse consequences which they attempted to reduce through precautions such as differentiation of safer and more dangerous situations, as illustrated above. The next quotation documents this approach to risk management.

> *Interviewer:* How do you feel about him going out on his own?

Mother: Well, he seems to enjoy it, but I worry about him until he comes in.

Interviewer: What type of thing do you worry about?

Mother: Is he still in the place, and is he wandering all over? (Heyman *et al.* 1998: 206)

As far as could be assessed within a qualitative study, differences in risk acceptance appeared unrelated to degree of disability, but was closely associated with socio-economic status, with better off families more likely to be risk-averse.

In only two of the twenty families was there a marked disagreement between the main family carer and the adult with learning disabilities about risk management. Such disagreements arose, in both cases, because the adult with learning disabilities aspired to, and judged himself capable of, managing more autonomy, for example, in relation to independent living. In both families, this difference in perspective generated intense interpersonal conflict. One adult with learning disabilities had abandoned his aspirations in order to keep the peace.

Interviewer: Do you ever still think about leaving the [day] centre?

Adult with learning disabilities: No. I am quite sorted, and I am quite happy with what I do. I shut up now. I can't change anything. Mum won't listen. It causes so much trouble that I don't say anything. (Heyman and Huckle 1995: 175)

Our research did not explore systematically the views of different family carers. But a similar phenomenon of a divergence of views about risk management generating interpersonal conflict, was observed in the case of a day centre manager who also became a service user when his own child was born with learning disabilities. He maintained his professional pro-risk attitude which was strongly opposed by his wife, generating intense interpersonal conflict. Experiences of 'crossing the floor', a service provider becoming a service user, can be instructive, showing up gaps in perspective between the two parties. More generally, such exceptional cases of overt conflict document the predication of interpersonal harmony on taken-for-granted shared attitudes towards risk.

Consideration of family risk management raises delicate issues about human rights versus political realities. For example, our research showed that some general practitioners routinely send out calls for cervical screening to families whom they know will discard them on the grounds that their daughter is not sexually active and, therefore, at very low risk of cervical cancer (Heyman *et al.* 2004). The doctors argued that the woman in question had the right to decide for herself whether to accept screening. However, in practice, the decision was made by parents. The right of women who could understand the issue to make their own decisions might have been better served if the GP had been able to engage the family in a discussion about screening. But this would have required an investment of time, a scarce health service resource, as noted above.

Decision-making power will not be split equally between adults with learning disabilities and carers on whom they depend. However, human relationships always involve an element at least of negotiation. Some adults with learning disabilities manage to persuade carers to support a more risk-accepting approach to their daily lives which yields gains in autonomy.

> *Family carer:* Well, I think he has achieved a lot more, despite my efforts to stop him. He's achieved a lot more than I thought he would. I never ever visualised him travelling on his own, going on the Metro on his own, even having a job. It's just been sheer determination and willpower on his part. (Heyman *et al.* 1998: 207–208)

Conclusion

This chapter has discussed risk management for adults with learning disabilities, with analysis centred around the efforts of risk managers (adults with learning disabilities, family and paid carers) to find an optimal balance between safety and autonomy. These parties have been described as risk managers in order to suggest that all are engaged in assessing and deciding about risks, however informally. We have seen that informal risk assessments can generate quite variable decision making, even in the same domain, for example, in relation to personal mobility. The views which adults with learning disabilities and carers take about risk taking, depend as much on their attitudes towards risks as they do on their assessment of the capabilities of the person with learning disabilities.

Quality of life for people with learning disabilities is very much affected by the degree of autonomy which they can exercise in their own lives. Depending on their abilities and aspirations, adults with learning disabilities may wish to live independently, to maintain employment or to visit friends on their own. Such autonomy has obvious benefits in terms of quality of life, mental health and provision of opportunities to develop new skills. However, these benefits have to be balanced against costs in terms of reduced safety and increased anxiety. Professional carers sometimes fail to acknowledge these costs (Alaszewski and Alaszewski 2002) particularly if risks occur outside their zone of accountability. Nurses and other caring professionals can support adults with learning disabilities and their carers in their efforts to find the best safety/autonomy balance for them if they can understand their risk concerns. Nurses who are called on to affirm *'dignity of risk'* (Shirtliffe 1995) should not create a tyranny of risk.

9 Balancing risk and independence in nursing older adults

Khim Horton

Introduction

Though risk is a key concern and preoccupation for both nurses and the older adults they care for, as Adams (1995) points out, it should be acknowledged that there are generational differences in how risk is perceived, with younger people more than older people being attuned to the debate on risk. Nurses, attuned to averting risks in the care of their patients, may forget that risks are often accompanied with rewards. For instance, when an older adult takes him/herself to the toilet, even though s/he may be at risk of falling, s/he has much to gain from his/her own independence. S/he is rewarded with the privacy that s/he would otherwise lose if s/he has to use a commode in a hospital bay, at the same time retaining his/her independence. Therefore, it is important that nurses are aware of such differences in risk perception and risk taking.

'Risk taking' has been defined as 'pursuing a course of action in order to realise one or more beneficial outcomes, in the knowledge that there are consequences or outcomes that would be perceived as negative or harmful in nature should they occur' (Saunders 1998: 75). Whatever happens, it is important to ensure that nurses put risk and risk taking into a therapeutic context, where the focus is on achieving realistic goals that are set in partnership with the older adult. This includes making sure that possibly harmful consequences are identified and reviewed in line with the changing circumstances of the older person.

The *National Service Framework for Older People* (Department of Health (DoH) 2001a) emphasises the need for increased user-participation, and for older adults to be involved in service evaluation, asserting the need for 'fair, high quality, integrated health and social care services for older people' (DoH 2001a: 1). The *National Service Framework* (NSF) also talks of the need to develop services that will support independence, avoiding unnecessary hospital admission, and ensuring speedy recovery and rehabilitation. In a quality of life study, Gabriel and Bowling (2004) demonstrate how older people place a high value on independence, as they perceive being able to walk and get about as crucially important, fearing loss of independence through poor health and immobility.

From the nurse's perspective, older adults are often identified as 'at risk', with those living alone being especially vulnerable to the power of the expert. Pickering and Thompson (1998) suggest that, inadvertently, nurses can easily be swept along by what is deemed to be 'for the best', with decisions which are made without informed consent from the client or significant other person. Often, nursing care plans indicate that an older adult is 'at risk' of developing pressure sores, a chest infection, and/or is at risk of falling. The Royal College of Nursing (RCN) (2004) suggests that there might be a temptation on the part of nurses to 'actively discourage' older adults from taking risks, to protect them from the risk of injury. This can often give rise to conflict with the older person's wishes.

Current research on risk and risk taking among older adults

Key issues raised in current research on risk and risk taking can provide a helpful insight into the way older adults perceive and take risks. Grinyer contended that 'to assume that risk to health could be separated from social risks, would be to minimise the complexity of the response to information about risk' (1995: 42). Individuals may weigh the social risks against perceived health risks, in order to decide which is deemed the lesser of two evils. Thus, older adults may be reluctant to inform their family members or friends about their health and/or social problems. Kingston (1998) found 87 of the 107 older adults in his study sample had not discussed falls they had suffered, either with their family members or with a friend. A phenomenological study of the experiences of older widows living alone at home suggests reasons for such behaviour (Porter 1994). Research subjects described how they 'avoided the need to intrude on their children or grandchildren for help' (Porter 1994: 121). This may explain why older adults are hesitant about seeking help from their children, or disclosing their need for help.

The risk of falling in older adults

The medical perspective of risk in caring for older adults tends to focus on pathological aspects of ageing. For example, Bennet and Ebrahim (1995) explain how changes in eyesight, such as reduction in acuity, or changes in mobility status, can place older adults at greater risk of falling because of their inability to manage hazards related to the environment. However, this dominant biomedical perspective provides a narrow understanding of the risk perceptions of falls. Amongst older adults the risk of falling is well documented. The risk of experiencing a fall increases during the retirement decades, with those in the oldest age group, 85 and over, being at greatest risk of falling (Dowswell *et al.*, 1999; Lord *et al.* 2001). Hip fractures resulting from falls are shown to occur in around 1 per cent of older adults who live in the community (Ballinger and Payne 2002). Older people with cognitive impairment and dementia are at greater risk of falls, with an annual incidence of about 60 per cent (Shaw *et al.* 2003).

Most commonly reported injuries resulting from falls include superficial cuts and bruises, abrasions, and sprains (Lord *et al.* 2001). Injuries from falling result in significant costs to health and social care services, a loss of independence for older adults and a reduced quality of life (Lord *et al.* 2001). The psychological impact from falls includes a fear of falling again (Horton and Arber 2004; Tinetti and Powell 1993), and withdrawal from activities (Bath and Morgan 1999). It is, therefore, not surprising that the NSF aims 'to reduce the number of falls which result in serious injury and ensure effective treatment and rehabilitation for those who have fallen' (DoH 2001a: 76). To achieve this, Acute and Primary Care Trusts have been working collaboratively to meet the targets set in Standard Six of the NSF, with a specific focus on falls among older adults.

Older adults' and their family carers' perceptions of the risk of falling

The way in which we identify and treat risks in our lives is shaped by a multitude of social factors. My own PhD study reveals some interesting gender-related variations in how the risk of falling is perceived by older adults and their family carers (Horton 2002). The study involved 40 interviews with older adults (20 men and 20 women) who were known for suffering recurrent falls. A further 35 family carers of these older adults were interviewed separately. The study found that reflective accounts of older adults about what caused them to fall revealed their perceptions and expectations of themselves and others. Older men in particular, portrayed themselves as 'responsible' and 'rational' individuals, as the following excerpt illustrate:

> *Mr Tibbs (aged 92):* I don't deliberately put myself at risk you know. Certainly not at my age.
>
> *Interviewer:* What sort of risk did you have in mind when you said you didn't deliberately put yourself at risk?
>
> *Mr Tibbs:* Oh anything that you shouldn't be doing if you know that's going to make you fall. Like if I know that getting up too soon will make me fall, then I jolly well make sure that I mustn't do that. I could hurt myself badly, then I would be no good to any one. I like to do as much as I can for myself.
>
> *Interviewer:* If you hurt yourself badly.
>
> *Mr Tibbs:* Yes, if I hurt myself badly, then I'll be needing more help from the district nurses. I might not be able to walk down again, who knows. (Horton 2002: 141)

Mr Tibbs sees the rational need to avoid doing things that can jeopardise his degree of independence. His desire to protect his own independence and autonomy can be seen through his deliberate and careful analysis of how he ought to get up slowly. Wynne-Harley (1991) similarly found, in their study, that maintenance of independence and autonomy influences the way older adults set limits and restrictions upon themselves.

Whilst most of the older men in my study saw themselves as rational and responsible, older women were more likely to be critical of those who took risks, blaming themselves and other older women for their falls:

> *Mrs Crick (aged 75):* A lady upstairs [in sheltered housing] goes round with a zimmer frame but you wouldn't think there was room in these houses. You have to think of things like having too much furniture when you're old, and having a microwave to heat your food. I have a friend who fell off a chair and broke her arm. She was stupid to go on the chair.
>
> *Interviewer:* Why was it stupid?
>
> *Mrs Crick:* Cleaning windows [laughs]. Oh no, not a chair, no. When my husband was alive he bought me a little step ladder to clean the windows, but it had handles on the side. But I would never dream of getting on a chair to clean my windows. (Horton 2002: 144)
>
> *Mrs Dench (aged 94):* There's a lady in this block of flats. She keeps falling, always ends up in hospital. She lives downstairs. Do you know, she still gets about with her sticks, silly really. I think she shouldn't be walking about like that, she's bound to fall. No wonder she keeps falling. She should be in a wheelchair really. (Horton 2002: 144)

How do we, as nurses, make sense of these accounts? They suggest that older adults consider themselves to be self-reliant, which supports Beck's (1992) idea that in late modern risk society we are all considered largely responsible for our own fate. Because Mrs Dench's neighbour chose to walk with sticks instead of using a wheelchair, Mrs Dench perceived her as being responsible for her frequent falls. What these accounts also show is the gendered meaning of the risk of falling: older men perceived themselves to be 'rational individuals' to legitimise their falls since their experiences were found to be more discrediting (Horton 2002). The blame apportioned by some of the older women to themselves and others also reflects what Douglas (1992) describes as risk operating as a 'forensic device', through which blame can be apportioned. However, these decisions were not always thought 'sound' in the eyes of the key family carers whom I interviewed. As in Manthorpe and Alaszewski's (2000) study, I also found that potentially negative consequences often influenced the risk perception of family carers, who considered their older relatives' quest for independence a risk factor for falls. Family carers believed certain domestic activities put the older adult at risk, as illustrated here by a daughter talking about her mother:

> There are certain things that I know I wouldn't do if I was at mum's age. It's just commonsense. It's simple tasks like vacuuming. I mean, she could have waited till I go round at weekends to do it for her but she still thinks she could do it. I do worry about it sometimes, in case she trips over the wire. It's just too much of a risk. But I know she likes to stay as independent as possible, but there are times when she's got to realise she can't any more. (Horton 2002: 154)

The desire to remain independent can place an older person at odds with family members. Porter found that widows often reported their children giving 'unsolicited precautionary advice or directions' such as you 'shouldn't be doing that [lawnmowing] anymore' (1994: 59). The notion that older people may be exposing themselves to risk, 'doing too much', can be contentious within the family when the older parent and their adult children have opposing perceptions about how much was too much. Thus, in accordance with the cultural approach of Douglas (1992), it can also be argued that these older adults and their family carers each culturally select the risks they attend to and those they ignore, according to that which each cares most about.

Risk and independence in hospital care setting for older adults

Falls among patients is a key concern within hospitals (Lord *et al.* 2001). Up to a quarter of patients, and up to 40 per cent of stroke patients fall during their time in hospital (Nyberg and Gustafson 1995). It is one of many risks that older people are particularly prone to when in hospital. Though the NSF (DoH 2001a) advocates that older adults should be beneficially treated in hospital, a multitude of risks militate against this desired outcome. As Masterson (1999) points out, older adults' multiple pathology, chronic illnesses and their compromised immune system, expose them to greater risk of developing complications within hospital, such as infection, confusion, incontinence and falls.

With regard to falls, there is, as Procter (2002) explains, a dynamic tension between risk and safety in the care of older adults. How do nurses decide when an older adult is safe to walk unaided, when they know the patient is at risk of falling? it is difficult to determine what could be considered an acceptable rate of falls within an acute care setting, since much depends on the profile of the in-patient population. Relative importance is attached to identifying key predictors of falls. Oliver *et al.* (1997) developed STRATIFY which involved an assessment of falls, transfer and mobility skills, patient agitation, the need for frequent toileting, and visual impairment. Their findings indicate that easily administered assessment tools can be useful in identifying those at risk of falling while in hospital.

However, though STRATIFY may be used successfully to reduce the alarming number of falls in hospital it is, perhaps, a quick solution to this urgent problem that pays little attention to the individual needs of older people. One might hope that the limitations of STRATIFY, and other such purely safety-focused approaches, might be more easily recognised beyond the hospital setting of acute care wards. Procter (2002) argues that in rehabilitation settings, where the aim is to minimise long-term disability in older adults, health care professionals are required to reduce patient dependency and increase autonomy during recovery. Therefore, over-protectiveness, and overt physical restraints and medical sedation are to be discouraged. Yet, as Hughes (2002) points out, organisation-centred processes in fall prevention tend to focus on the monitoring of falls and the use of fall risk assessment, with little emphasis on how to improve the older person's balance, strength or flexibility problems.

In a care setting, such as a day hospital for older adults, the provision of a safe environment to keep risks at a minimum is as important as it is in a hospital setting. In their ethnographical study, Ballinger and Payne (2002) described ways in which risk was realised and managed in a day hospital for older adults. From participant observation and semi-structured interviews discourse analysis was used to examine these issues with staff and 15 attendees. The researchers found that attendees were most concerned with the risk to their personal and social identities, expressing concern about being infantilised and stereotyped in interpersonal exchanges. In contrast, service providers were most concerned about the management of physical risk. This illustrates why care professionals need to adopt a person-centred approach and value the personal contribution of an older person. There is a need to recognise that for some older adults, hospitalisation presents a traumatic event in their life, in which their hold on independent living becomes tenuous.

Ballinger and Payne's (2000) study indicates that the day centre staff perceived older adults as being ignorant of danger, which rendered them vulnerable. For example, a therapist described how she regarded an older woman's rejection of a Lifeline pendant as a rejection of good advice and a challenge to her authority, without consideration of any alternative perspectives of risk and safety that the older woman may have had. The therapist portrayed the older woman as 'foolhardy and not acting in her best interests' (Ballinger and Payne 2002: 576). Invariably, patient decisions and behaviour were also cited as contributing to the likelihood of a fall. However, from the older adult's perspective, the construction of the meaning of the risk of falling suggests that bad luck or the incompetence of others contributed to falls. Most of the older adults in this study reported themselves able to manage at home, if not independently, then with readily available help.

Procter describes the more positive work of a nursing development unit, which focused on the whole area of risk taking, and 'the delicate balance between promoting activity and independence, and protecting patients from harm' (2002: 55). She explains how, in promoting an environment that is both stimulating and 'open', the nurses recognised that some patients may sustain falls. Procter draws particular attention to the need to fully engage in dialogue with patients and relatives relating to the risks and costs to quality of life, and over-protection.

Balancing risk and independence in the primary care settings

Living independently can become a major issue when health-related factors impact on an older person. To determine when an older adult is safe to live alone, against their desire to live independently, poses a challenge for nurses when they encounter an older person deemed 'at risk'. For some older adults, the benefits of being considered as an active, relatively independent person, may outweigh the risk of falls. Some take risks in an active lifestyle, asserting their independence, whilst others lead a more restrictive, risk-averse lifestyle, fearing the post-fall trajectory of - hospital, nursing home and death.

Denscombe (1993: 507) indicated that perceptions of the extent of risk are crucially affected by the 'dread factor', the vividness of the risk, the frequency with which the risk is encountered, the 'sense of invulnerability', and the 'tendency to dismiss low risks as negligible and not worth worrying about'. Denscombe maintained that the dread factor influences perceptions in relation to the level of risk posed by a particular threat. How vivid a risk is, can be influenced by two salient factors: personal experience and exposure to information. In other words, the more frequently an individual is confronted with information concerning a specific risk, the less serious the individual regards the risk. Where people are exposed to a risk frequently the evidence is that they tend to perceive the risk as less likely to happen than they would if they were exposed to the risk only occasionally. The more regular and routine is the exposure of the risk, the lower is the expectation that the risk 'could happen to me' (Denscombe 1993: 507).

At home, the familiar presence of rugs in their home can lead older adults to have a lower expectation that the risk of tripping on rugs could happen to them. In my own study, older adults living in the community rarely identified hazards within their home as something that might cause them to fall (Horton 2002).

Contrary to health care professionals' understanding, Clemson et al. (1996) found the homes of 'fallers' were no more hazardous than the homes of non-fallers. Yet environmental modifications or removal of environmental hazards are major fall-prevention strategies employed by health care professionals. Though compliance with such measures can be difficult, early studies (Gosselin *et al.* 1993) indicate that only a small percentage of people failed to follow advice about environmental modifications. Ryan and Spellbring (1996) found that advice is least taken when nurses recommend removing rugs or the relocation of furniture. Although many older people know what could, in general terms, be done to prevent falls they do not modify their homes to make them safer (Carter *et al.* 1997; Clemson *et al.* 1999). In Carter's cross-sectional interview survey of 425 people, 97 per cent of those aged 70 and over rated their home as fairly safe or very safe. However, those who were never seen by service providers were far more likely to have home hazards than those who were visited regularly. This offers insight into how older people perceive the safety of their home environment, and how recognition of home hazards is not necessarily conducive to action to make their homes safer.

'Trade-offs'

The decision to move from living independently to living with family members or within an assisted housing scheme remains a difficult one for older adults as they attempt to balance risk and independence. This has sometimes led to their reluctance to visit their GP after a fall or an accident in case they were considered 'at risk' and in need of nursing or therapeutic interventions.

A study, commissioned by the Department of Trade and Industry Consumer Safety Unit (Wynne-Harley 1991), investigating the extent to which older adults consciously accepted or incorporated risks in their daily lives, found that most interviewees saw risk to themselves mainly in terms of falls, consequent fractures (of the femur), burns (or fires) from domestic appliances, and hypothermia: sometimes a direct result of a fall and lack of immediate attention. It was also found that older adults managed these risks by balancing multiple costs and benefits. As Reed (1998) points out, they may accept certain risks in order to avoid being patronised by professionals or younger relatives. Wynne-Harley (1991) also illustrates how older adults 'trade-off' certain risks. She cited an example of a woman who was more concerned about the risk of dying of hypothermia, if she fell in an unheated bathroom, than being electrocuted and tripping over wires. In another example, a woman continued to use her bicycle to alleviate her arthritis, which she regards as a major threat to her quality of life, worse than that of being involved in a road traffic accident. Most older adults choose to continue to live alone rather than move to a nursing or residential home, despite acknowledging they are at a greater risk of having falls if they remain in their own home.

The aim of balancing risk and independence may become less clear where managing care with those who are cognitively frail are concerned. Miesen (1995) argues that to exclude people with dementia from active participation in their care is to 'metaphorically decapitate' them. Studies have shown that highly impaired older adults living in the community were passive for much of their waking lives, with only 7 per cent of their time spent in what they termed 'potentially enriching activity' (Lawton et al. 1995). This suggests that by maintaining and/or encouraging passivity, health care professionals can indirectly 'restrain' older adults from undertaking activities that might put them at risk. Dewing (1999) argues that as people with dementia do not generally act in a way that puts them at risk, it is the nurses who accentuate the problem by misinterpreting the meaning of patient behaviour. Therefore, the challenge to nurses is for them to have a proper understanding of patient behaviour, and to recognise the need to provide enriching stimulation for all older adults, in all community and institutional care settings.

Risk and care home settings

Like other care settings, nurses in care homes are placed in an awkward and difficult position. Redfern and Ross (1999) assert that the dignity and rights of service users is of paramount importance, particularly where balancing the risk of accident against the dignity and rights of service users. To maximise their independence, nursing staff need to empower their service users to be proactive, by offering genuine choice, and opening access to the outside world. However, the fear of recrimination, in case an accident happens, might lead nurses to resort to restricting the service user, for example, by confining him/her to bed during the night. In fall-prevention programmes, staff in care homes pay particular attention to environmental modifications, by reducing hazards in the common areas (Jensen *et al.* 2003).

Keeping older adults physically active is an important care aspect, in line with the Care Home Standards criteria (DoH 2001b). Nevertheless, staff may be reluctant to instigate physical activities to improve stability and balance, lest that an older user could fall and/or sustain physical injury. The risk perceptions of health professionals can, therefore, influence the manner in which person-centred care is delivered and managed.

Conclusion

An understanding of the construction of risk by older adults would enable nurses to reveal that it is commonly constructed as a challenge to a person's self-image and identity. This understanding explains the responses of older adults to complex health problems and to the services and treatments employed to solve them. As Ballinger and Payne (2002) point out, these responses may sometimes mean that older adults 'trade-off' in order to maintain their independence. Though Pickering and Thompson (1999) alert us to the reluctance of some older adults in making choices about whether to take risks or not, which should be acknowledged and accepted. What is crucially important is the opportunity for older adults to have a say in the decision-making process relating to any aspect of their care.

Caring for older adults frequently requires an approach that is collaborative, multi-disciplinary, and inter-agency. With respect to risk taking in professional practice, the only way forward may be to bend or break existing rules to adopt an unorthodox approach in order to achieve an outcome that is person-centred. It is likely, therefore, that nurses will have to learn to be creative and willing to take a risk if the outcome is likely to enhance health promotion and the well-being of the older adult. Lloyd (2004) asserts that nurses should be reminded that, at the individual level, older adults are acutely aware of the risks inherent in being seen to have become 'decrepit'. Minichiello *et al.* (2000) suggested that in contemporary western societies, increased dependency is inextricably linked with the loss of autonomy. Discussion about risk assessment often ignores the point of view of the older adult involvement. This can result in paternalistic judgements about what is right for someone else; for, as Grinyer (1995) points out, there is the unwillingness, not least amongst professionals, to recognise lay knowledge.

There is a danger that paternalistic and rigid approaches adopted by nurses in relation to their notions of risk and risk taking can lead to a detached appreciation of the needs of older adults to maintain their independence. Yet, authoritative voices from within nursing call for a more balanced approach. The RCN (2004) states that professional responsibility of nurses includes risk taking, which entails them attaining a point where benefits outweigh potential harms. Saunders (1988) asserts that it is essential for nurses to realise that they can work with older adults and their families and/or significant others to maximise benefits, whilst at the same time keeping risk at a tolerable level. In order for this to work, nurses need to acquire and apply knowledge and understanding of the social context of risk and risk taking.

10 Managing risk – the case of sexualities and sexual health

Anthony Pryce

Introduction

Sex is risky, not just in terms of disease or unwanted pregnancy but in the social conduct of individuals and populations. Historically, sexuality represents risks that are private and public: troublesome and dangerous to institutional religions and the State. Socially, sexual conduct is predicated on laws and regulation through codes of shame, taboo, honour and propriety whilst individually driven by powerful, embodied and sometimes apparently irrational desires. No other arena of human rationality and conduct is more vulnerable and yet elusive to control than sexuality. This is particularly so where the individual may disregard risk or reconstruct it as a pleasurable, even as the defining element in the pursuit of erotic desire such as forms of fetishism, exhibitionism and voyeurism (such as 'dogging') or voluntary unprotected sex ('barebacking').

In this chapter, I shall consider the constructions of sexuality and sexual health risk and its management by the individual in contemporary cultures. This clearly has an impact on the way nurses and other health care professionals think about sex, sexualities and health. The appropriate management of sexuality is problematic for people and is largely dependent on the successful performance of their roles in their interactions with others in everyday life. Simon and Gagnon originated the notion that individuals employ 'scripts' which are 'a metaphor for conceptualising the production of behaviour in social life' (1999: 29). In other words, such scripts provide the working basis for the performance of the individual's gendered and sexual role, consistent with the demands and expectations of identity and desire within a particular culture. Drawing, in part, on this notion of 'sexual scripting', sexual behaviour can be conceptualised in three key domains:

1. Collective and cultural meanings of sex, the erotic and its regulation;
2. The interpersonal, 'capillary-level' conduct of sexual practices;
3. Individual, or intrapsychic, fantasy and symbolic constructions of the self and sexual identity;

to which we can add here,

4. the biological consequences of sex such as (unwanted) pregnancy and sexually acquired infections (SAI's). (A domain with which of course health care professions are particularly concerned.)

These each represent historical continuities, for example the biological consequences of sex being disease or unwanted pregnancy have always been problematic. However, each of these four domains is continuously reconstructed in the light of contemporary discourses and the invention of 'new' populations organised around sexual identities, for instance gay men, transgender, or the emergence of moral panics such as that around paedophilia. As I will show, sexuality has been increasingly problematised and contemporary technologies reflect (or even drive) the post-modern *vibe* of erotic consumption, the ideal of self-actualisation and the formation of an 'authentic' sexual identity central to the individual's 'project of the self'. This 'vibe' resonates with the tensions between social controls and private individual freedoms, the 'right' of self-expression and sexual experimentation through neo-liberal economies of consumption such as porn or Internet sex chat rooms. The rapid increase in the access and use of the Internet demonstrates how some of these tensions operate within sexual health discourses and the population(s) and practices that are identified as 'risky'. I shall, therefore, consider the notion of sexual health as a discursive element in policy formation and the behavioural and epidemiological factors that continually resurface as troublesome signifiers of risk. I will draw on both Douglas's (1966) notion of purity and danger, and Foucault to demonstrate how the individual as a monitoring agent of his or her own sexual practices, is recruited to become the self-monitoring overseer 'or active patient' (Armstrong 1995;

Pryce 2000). In so doing, the individual is alerted to their own 'conduct of conduct', or in other words becomes deployed within a network of (self) surveillance that works as a means of governmentality in the management of their sexual careers, practices and the calculation of sex risks.

I will first consider sexual health risks posed by increases in Sexually Acquired Infections (SAI's) and other risk factors. It is important to contextualise this somewhat, and consider what is meant by sexuality and how contemporary technologies are affecting sexual practices, beliefs and opportunities for new identities. These changes create or heighten risks and I will provide brief illustrations of the relationship between the imperative, or drive, of risk and some new constructions of sex. Second, I will suggest how Internet sex chat rooms are providing arenas for individuals to rehearse ideas, desires and practices online that they may go on to enact offline. These activities may represent transgressive forces that are contributing to the destabilising of sexual categories and sexual identities such as 'straight', 'gay', 'bisexual' and so on, as well as the production of a wider menu of erotic practices available to the individual to explore.

I will conclude with some consideration of how these 'new' phenomena fit with earlier formations of sexual risk and the contemporary rubrics of sexual citizenship and the operation of governmentality in everyday life. These clearly have significant implications for the defining and management of sexual risk by clinical professionals who are themselves, of course, individuals engaged in the project of sexuality.

Risky sex

Before addressing risk, it is helpful to consider how sex and sexualities can be explained as problematic sites of danger and threat. The theory and practice of sex and sexuality is enmeshed in complex relationships of one form or another, and as Foucault conceptualised it, sex

> appears rather as an especially dense transfer point for relations of power: between men and women, young people and old people, parents and offspring, teachers and students, priests and laity, an administration and a population. (1978: 103)

Certainly, this renders sex a most powerful and pervasive element in human activities. Power is critical in relations such as those between doctors, nurses and patients; and where sexuality is both the clinical subject and a potential interactional danger, the instrumentality of sexuality produces new combinations of risk. Foucault argued that power operated at the 'capillary', or individual, level and that it

> reaches into the very grain of individuals, touches their bodies and inserts itself into their actions and attitudes, their discourses, learning processes and everyday lives. (1980: 30)

It can be argued that the performance of sexual identities, erotic practices and interactions echoes this, and provides the basis for deeply engrained and taken-for-granted assumptions of gendered roles and sexual orientation as 'natural' or 'unnatural'. As both a vector of disease and as social agency, sexuality has long been engaged in a discursive tension with medicine. Sex has been pathologised as bio-psycho-social danger in itself, whilst also constructed as a downright threat to the conduct of professional healthcare where any suggestion of sexual expression by clients or practitioners is deeply subversive and transgressive. Foucault argues sexuality is

> not the most intractable element in power relations, but rather one of those endowed with the greatest instrumentality: useful for the greatest number of manoeuvres and capable of serving as a point of support, as a lynchpin, for the most varied strategies. (1978: 105)

This great surface network of power relations is the social world of everyday life where bodies interact physically and symbolically, each individual potentially the object of desire but also the subject of propriety laws, taboos, forms of knowledge (such as medicine) and moral order. Douglas (1976) provided a powerful analysis of how all societies operate to control the threat of pollution or impurity through the notion of 'dirt as matter out of place' (1966: 35). Of course we are familiar with numerous ways in which part of the body and bodily functions are almost universally regarded and dirty, contaminated or dangerous. These processes, activities of embodiment itself carry a heavy symbolic load and where some actions, objects or activities may be regarded as 'clean' or 'pure', and others signify dirt, contamination and impurity. It implies two conditions: a set of ordered social relations and a contravention of that order. According to Douglas, dirt or pollution is never a

> unique, isolated event and where there is dirt there is a system; it is the by-product of a systematic ordering and classification of matter, in so far as ordering involves rejecting inappropriate elements. (1966: 35)

In everyday life, Douglas argues that

> In chasing dirt, in papering, decorating, tidying, we are not governed by anxiety to escape disease, but are positively re-ordering our environment, making it conform to an ideal. (1966: 2)

Similarly, human sexuality and desire represents a huge project of control and order because of its destabilising effect on individuals, communities and beliefs. If dirt (or unregulated sexuality) is matter out of place, it must is controlled through social and moral order as dirt is that which must not be included if a pattern is to be maintained. The same principle applies throughout history and all societies because, as Douglas asserts 'it involves no special distinction between primitives and moderns: we are all subject to the same rules' (1966: 40).

Godin, in Chapter 1, has already explored Douglas's (1992) notion of the grid/group model to explain how different understandings and meanings are given to risk. In the same way, sex and sexuality occupy zones of cultural and individual threat, especially from people at the borders of society, or on the boundaries between social or sexual categories that are perceived as possessing both power and danger. For example, the status of the 'bisexual' is contested and a threat because, as Esterberg (2002) suggests, its status remains unclear and challenges deeply held assumptions of the 'natural' or 'essential' notion of sexual orientation and practices.

> What is bisexuality? Is it an identity that a person holds, something one *is*? Is it a behavior, something one *does*? Is it stable, or does it shift and float and change? Is bisexuality distinct from heterosexuality and homosexuality? Is it a bit of both and neither? Does bisexuality disrupt the dichotomous way in which we are used to thinking about sexuality? (One is either straight *or* gay). (2002: 215)

Thus, bisexuals, transgendered individuals and other groups might be constructed as dangerous, subversive and destabilising threats to 'normal', 'pure' sexual categories and practices. In all societies we may find a rule against contact with the marginal person or thing especially where there is great symbolic meaning and risk such as sexual intercourse, pregnancy, birth and death exist at the border between different stages of life, and all are frequently surrounded by taboos. Thus, it is not just the body that may be 'dirty', but what the body signifies in terms of potential or actual pollution, such as masturbation or other erotic practices conducted either alone or with others, where sexual deeds (and even thoughts) are constructed as dirty, sinful, contaminating and must be confessed and controlled within the moral order of society. To challenge, subvert or contravene the taboos and conventions that maintain order is to render individual sexual activity as not just a 'bad' behaviour but represent a 'type' – a spoiled identity as 'dirty pervert' or 'filthy degenerate' acting outside the sanitary conditions of 'pure' state such as virginity or union sanctified through marriage.

Douglas's ideas here might be interpreted as overly deterministic and structured, maybe insufficiently geared to reflect contemporary, more 'liberal' expectations in contemporary life. Jeffrey Weeks (2000) argued that newer understandings of sexual history have challenged the notion of 'the natural', have deconstructed sexuality so that it may be reconstructed, whilst recognising and coming to terms with the moral and sexual diversity of the past and the present. However, ideas of hygiene, sanitation and the ideal of 'natural' purity have seldom been more pervasive than in twenty-first century culture. Here the emphasis is on knowledge and self-regulation of body management and the post-AIDS hygiene ideologies around safer sex and the management of pleasure on the one hand, and discourses of pre-marital celibacy on the other. Both Douglas (1992) and Sontag (1988) highlight the tendency for victim blaming in response to contagion, such as AIDS. It seems that notions of sexual purity, the contamination of dangerous sexual 'otherness', disgust and the potential defiling quality of body fluids and the virtues of sexual and social hygiene remain as powerful, if not more so now, as in any other earlier period of history.

The conventional ideas of the history of sexuality suggests that there was a 'golden age' of emotional and physical expression that was then systematically repressed through moralising forces in bourgeois society and the increasing management of the individual's erotic behaviour. Foucault, however, rejects this notion and offers a working hypothesis that nineteenth-century society did not repress sex, but on the contrary

> Not only did it speak of sex and compel everyone to do so; it set out to formulate the uniform truth of sex. As if it suspected sex of harbouring a fundamental secret. As if it needed this production of truth. As if it was essential that sex be inscribed not only in an economy of pleasure but in an ordered system of knowledge. (1978: 69)

The machinery of this 'system' was not only the development of forms of knowledge like sexology, psychology and clinical practices such as psychoanalysis, but also the organisation of the family in its structure and roles. According to Foucault (1978) the family in the nineteenth century became the object of surveillance, a panoptic site where four key *strategic unities* provided the basis for

- Malthusian organisation of heterosexual, monogamous marriage and the family as the basic unit of capitalist society;
- Intensification of medico-moral discourses that located woman not only as emotionally and physically unstable but also 'hysterical';
- Pathologising and criminalising of 'perverse' or unorthodox erotic pleasure and non-heteronormative sex;
- The social construction of childhood innocence and heightened anxieties about sex, masturbation and the young.

Foucault argues that these 'strategic unities' lie at the heart of notions of sexual and gendered relations and underpinned the recruitment of the individual into the project of self-monitoring surveillance and governmentality, or the 'conduct of conduct' as a term which Lemke interprets as ranging from 'governing the self' to 'governing others' (2001: 191). These techniques of governmentality were produced and reproduced in bodies of knowledge constructed through modernist scientific, social and moral discourses of the nineteenth and twentieth centuries. Those earlier procedures were central to ancient cultures such as Rome, Greece or India, where individual (male) sexuality is

rooted in the knowledge (Ars Erotica) gained from the refine-
ment of the individual's own experience of erotic pleasure or
'askēsis'.

'Askēsis', according to Foucault, presents the possibility for
the individual to enjoy types of sexual pleasure without reference to 'exterior law of the permitted and the forbidden, ... but first and foremost in relation to itself' (1978: 57).
For example, whilst Greek and Roman men may have engaged
in same sex activities, it was only acceptable within conventional notions of power. In other words, an older man might
have sex with a younger man but only if he played the 'active'
role, as to do otherwise would be to usurp their hierarchical
power relations (Constantinos 2003). This remains the case in
many contemporary, patriarchal cultures such as those in the
Mediterranean and Middle East (Faubion 1993). Similarly,
the act of rape is often conceptualised more in terms of gender and power than sexual pleasure. Where a man has raped
other males this disruption to the 'natural' order of things is
even more apparent where penetration ceases to be about gendered or erotic power but appears as a profound threat to
socially constructed notions of masculinity and the stability
that is assumed to drive and control sexual orientation. Even
the implied or symbolic threat, particularly to hegemonic
notions of masculinity is regarded as an almost perpetual risk
that must be avoided through carefully coded rules of male
interaction and performativity.

The individual is engaged in the project of refining and
developing his or her appreciation of sexual pleasure. Civil
rights movements that have emerged over the last 50 years
reclaimed or created new identities which both politicise the
individual and the collective, such as the 'queer' and 'coming out'
as a rite of passage in the process of acquiring an 'authentic'
identity. Giddens (1992) argued that contemporary concerns
with rights, identity and the search for the 'authentic self' has
resulted in the self becoming for everyone a reflexive project
that is,

a more or less continuous interrogation of past, present and future. It
is a project carried on amid a profusion of reflexive resources: therapy
and self-help manuals of all kinds, television programmes and maga-
zine articles. (1992: 30)

In the period that has elapsed since Giddens wrote this, it is clear that further, accessible resources have included the Internet and the abundance of technologies and discourses that have located risk as a key component in the construction of the 'reflexive project' of sexual behaviours and identities of both the individual and populations. However, Giddens's comments remain relevant as he highlights the tensions between the ways in which the individual citizen is expected to engage with the self-monitoring of their inner world, secret and potentially stigmatising desires. However, despite being immersed in the incitement to the consumption of pleasure, the individual is bombarded with sometimes competing and conflicting information, ideologies and the re-construction of social values and attitudes. Not least among these conflicting influences is the role of public health that, as Coveney and Bunton suggest, attempts to transform carnal and embodied pleasure, but

> always runs the risk of introducing new and unanticipated elements that may run counter to the goals of health enhancement. In part, this is because it has not been able to theorize the place of pleasure in health and well-being. (2003: 174)

In increasingly globalising societies, the reality of an individual's sexual practices may lead to a dissonance in the tensions between embodied practices and expectations. For example, the media, through soap operas and the invention of celebrity cults, is simultaneously producing and reproducing new orthodoxies such as 'ideal' body types and the increasing accessibility of cosmetic surgery. However, the same media is engaged in the deployment of moral panic through risk discourses such as those around teenage pregnancies or paedophilia. The result of this has been that the child and children's bodies have been invested with danger to an observer, where even a parental hug or kiss may signify sexual risk, especially for men. A corresponding discourse has focused on the incitement to talk about actual or imagined sexual transgressions or stigmatising desire. Similarly, the expansion of self-help resources on the Internet and elsewhere is available for the individual who is increasingly expected to utilise these as a way of self-reliance and social responsibility. They can be seen as a means of negotiating the mire of risk that may engulf the unwary individual in daily life. Having said that, many nurses feel unprepared to engaged patients in confessional interactions of sexual behaviour, anxieties, values or lifestyle for fear that it might produce information for which they might be ill-equipped to successfully contain within their role. The potential 'erotic charge' between client and professional signifies a notion of pollution (Douglas 1966) so that in the clinic therefore, sex(uality) stays firmly within the clinical closet and controlled through the maintenance of symbolic sanitary ritual practices! Lawler (1991) describes how nurses accomplish 'body work', keeping sexual readings of interactions in check whilst washing and otherwise attending to naked bodies.

Few other areas in the conduct of the contemporary individual are so vulnerable to control through self-surveillance as sexuality, whilst few other components of human experience are as resistant to rationality as erotic desire and practices. Herein lies the problem for post-modern sexualities and the individual's management of sexuality and sexual health. Given the scepticism at the heart of the 'post-modern condition' (Lyotard 1979) it seems that 'grand narratives' such as religion, science, law or politics can no longer be a sufficient basis to simply ban or exclude or pathologise some sexual behaviours, orientations or identities. The civil rights movements of the twentieth century have produced (in some areas) an increasing tolerance even if not acceptance of sexual diversity and the legitimacy, albeit contested, of some sexual identities such a 'gay' or 'transgender'. Similarly, despite the impact of AIDS, the centrality of sexual identities and the ironic playfulness with which these may be taken on, such as gender bending or fetishism, has been mainstreamed.

Of course, what is mainstream in cool 'metrosexual'[1] (Simpson 1994) culture may be regarded with some hostility

---

[1] Mark Simpson originated the term 'Metrosexual in 1994. He later refined the definition: The typical **metrosexual** is a young man with money to spend, living in or within easy reach of a metropolis – because that's where all the best shops, clubs, gyms and hairdressers are. He might be officially gay, straight or bisexual, but this is utterly immaterial because he has clearly taken himself as his own love object and pleasure as his sexual preference. Particular professions, such as modeling, waiting tables, media, pop music and, nowadays, sport, seem to attract them but, truth be told, like male vanity products and herpes, they're pretty much everywhere – 'Meet the **metrosexual**,' *Salon.com*, July 22, 2002.

elsewhere, and the individual's calculation of sexual risk may need to include aggressive responses by others to overt violations of local social codes of heterosexuality. To challenge or subvert essentialist (usually patriarchal), heteronormative, sexual worldviews is often to create 'difference', the queer – the 'other' and thereby present a risk and threat to the 'moral' majority. Nevertheless, the heightened awareness of sexual diversity in erotic practices and social identity has been underscored by the use of the term 'sexualities' which itself carries a positive but challenging note of social (and sexual) inclusion and diversity. However, for the some who identify with the 'moral' majority, the emergence of sexual diversity and inclusion generates further social and sexual risk. It problematises conventional social arrangements and assumptions with grey areas of moral relativism, and the fear of subverting the status of the family is fuelling much contemporary discourse around legal recognition of the so-called gay *marriage*. In relation to contemporary gay culture, Foucault suggested that 'what bothers many heterosexuals about gayness is the implied sexual and interpersonal freedoms of the lifestyle, not sex acts themselves' (1989: 228). When he elaborated on this, Bristow (1997) suggested that Foucault's notion of 'genuine' forms of sexual freedom involved 'unforeseen', casual sexual relationships in public places and the complex exchanges of erotic power in S/M (sadomasochism) may be unintelligible to 'outsiders'. For the minority who take on the sexual identity of 'other', the risk is one of being oppressed and the danger of social and physical violence (usually) by men who feel compelled to patrol and control the boundaries of heteronormative masculinity.

Social policy – sexual practice

Social and individual calculations of risk relating to undesirable consequences of sexual activity have always been present in some form or other. A contemporary example is the response of the church to the widespread allegations of sexual abuse. Despite the imperative to purity and celibacy, several Catholic archdioceses in the United States of America (USA) face bankruptcy due to the great number of claims of sexual abuse by priests and the alleged collusion by the hierarchy who were insufficiently rigorous in reducing the risk to the young people in their care. Similarly, the trial of pop star Michael Jackson, was partly concerned with what constitutes sexual activity, abuse and how an observer might interpret behaviour.

Clearly, we have difficulty in some cases in actually defining what we mean by 'sexual' behaviour and of course an outside observer often may only guess at another person's erotic universe. Similarly, that sexual health requires a specific definition is important because it underscores the various ways that national and international policy has emerged to deal with the 'problem' of sexuality, sexual practices, public control and private freedoms in the context of an intensification of the medicalisation of sex since the nineteenth century. In so doing, of course, it has created a corresponding arena of new sexual risk. Giami (2002) provides an insightful historical analysis that reveals how emerging definitions of sexual health have focused on sexually acquired diseases and reproductive issues such as contraception, abortion or gender re-assignments (sex change) as risky problems. The emphasis on sexual rights, enshrined in the World Health Organization (WHO) Declaration of 1975, was central to the discourse at that time. While recognising that it is difficult to arrive at a universally acceptable definition of the totality of human sexuality, the following definition of sexual health is presented as a step in this direction:

> Sexual health is the integration of the somatic, emotional, intellectual, and social aspects of sexual being, in ways that are positively enriching and that enhance personality, communication, and love. Fundamental to this concept are the right to sexual information and the right to pleasure. (WHO 1975: 41)

The early WHO declaration stated that the concept of sexual health includes three basic elements:

1. a capacity to enjoy and control sexual and reproductive behavior in accordance with a social and personal ethic,
2. inhibiting sexual response and impairing sexual relationship,
3. freedom from organic disorders, diseases, and deficiencies that interfere with sexual and reproductive functions. (WHO 1975: 41)

Thus, the WHO notion of sexual health implies a positive approach to human sexuality, and the purpose of sexual health care should be the enhancement of life and personal relationships and not merely procreation or sexuality transmitted diseases. It must be remembered however, that this defining was constructed in a pre-AIDS period of liberationist optimism. The current working definition (WHO 2002) is now almost wholly predicated on sexual rights that embrace human rights already recognised in national laws, international human rights documents and other consensus documents

- the highest attainable standard of health in relation to sexuality, including access to sexual and reproductive health care services;
- seek, receive and impart information in relation to sexuality;
- sexuality education;
- choice of partner;
- consensual sexual relations;
- consensual marriage;
- pursue a satisfying, safe and pleasurable sexual life.

This list of sexual rights does provide the basic reference points that all individuals must negotiate in the conduct of their sexual career, and each presents a potential panorama of social and sexual risks. This WHO document concludes with the assertion that 'the responsible exercise of human rights requires that all persons respect the rights of others' (WHO 2002). However, this appears to assume a universal recognition of human rights and a consensus on moral values and socially acceptable gender/power relations. A number of problematic questions can arise from these assumptions. For example, what are the boundaries to consent and abuse? How emotionally or socially dangerous might it be for a hitherto 'straight' man or woman to contemplate having same sex experience? What freedom or power does the individual woman have in relation to fertility or choice of partner? What constitutes a pleasurable sexual life when one partner may have different sexual desires? What constitutes propriety in terms of sexual expression and the body? What forms of knowledge provide the basis for sex education? What is the moral and social status of sex work?

Whereas the United Kingdom (UK) government's *National Strategy on Sexual Health and HIV* (DoH 2002) is concerned with sexual health, it actually tends to focus on the negative consequences of unsafe sexual activity. It is constructed through highly medicalising strategies whilst also foregrounding the role of the individual in managing risk reduction. The United States (US) sexual health strategy document *The Surgeon General's Call To Action To Promote Sexual Health And Responsible Sexual Behavior* (Department of Health & Human Services 2001) on the other hand, reflects the current tensions that pervade North American cultural discourses that polarise liberal secular attitudes and the neo-conservative, religious-Right moral agenda. Giami argues that the *Call To Action* makes proposals that are 'not strictly part of the field of health but, rather, are aimed at the sexual activity' (2002: 32). As we have already seen in Chapter 1, herein lies the problem for the individual who is increasingly recruited into the project of self monitoring him/herself for compliance with the numerous indices of risk in everyday life, whether in relation to diet, lifestyle, drinking, smoking, ensuring optimum financial acumen in choice of bank/insurance/mortgage/pension or choice of car. Many of these issues are located in discourses of individual rights, consumerism, and (with individual fluency in risk management) as a 'moral' signifier of responsible citizenship. The individual is required to negotiate their sexual career in a culture that is saturated with sexual incitement, desire, spectacle and display, whilst conforming to prevailing conventions such as fidelity within monogamous, heterosexual relationships. The apparent loosening of sexual mores is, however, being supplanted by increasingly judgmental debates based on economic and moralising rationales, for instance, around prostitution and sex work. The question is now less concerned with the risk of becoming not respectable for having had sex, but whether the sexual activity was performed in a risky way.

A human cesspit of their own making – the construction of cultural risk

James Anderton, the former Chief Constable of Manchester, made this notorious comment when speaking at a press conference on AIDS in 1987. He was primarily referring to people with AIDS (and other conditions) infected as a result of sexual activities, and clearly locates the individual as the author of personal misfortune as a result of indulging immoral, carnal drives. In so doing, Anderton was drawing on ancient cultural histories that predicate transgressive sexual identities and erotic practices as impure and sinful. There are threats, in the form of diseases and other unwanted sequelae of sexual practices that form the basis of individual calculations of risk. As we have already noted from Douglas's work, disease and exclusion from 'respectable' society as a result of deviation whether by adultery or other taboo practices, has been a recurrent risk in virtually all societies. The reality and the risk to the individual is that sex is fraught with social, religious and biological danger. It is an event that is the core of the embodied human experience where bodily fluids such as menstrual blood carry massive symbolic load of potential danger and threat, particularly for men (Douglas 1966: 140). Particularly in affluent developed societies like the UK and US, the focus of anxiety remains on the continuing, alarming increase in the number of teenage pregnancies and the prevalence of SAI's.

The UK government set up an independent advisory group to focus on prevention of sexually transmitted infections. The group for Sexual Health and HIV called on the government to do more to reduce sexually transmitted infections by stripping away the stigma and making prevention a key part of the nation's broader public health agenda through the White Paper *Choosing Health?* (Department of Health: 2004). The Group claimed sexual health needed to become a mainstream issue, incorporated into other key public health initiatives.

Some believe sexual health issues to be shameful – a kind of Pandora's box of sins unleashed on a permissive society. It's time to destigmatise sexual health and deal with it properly in an adult fashion. (Gould 2004)

This 'adult fashion' is of course elusive in Judeo-Christian and other cultures where the body, and more particularly sexuality, remain highly problematic moral and social issues. It is clear that the UK policy was not only constructed around neo-liberal discourses of rights and progress, but also at the heart of the political economy of health. Concern, at the medical, economic and political policy level, is rising around the threat of SAIs. The Health Protection Agency (HPA) reported that cases of chlamydia, the most common sexually transmitted infection, had increased by 9 per cent. Sexually acquired infections (SAIs) and their complications cost in excess of £700 million per annum (HPA 2004). It is thought that complacency about condom use, increased numbers of sexual partners and long waits for treatment may all be helping to fuel the trend. The HPA Annual Report argued that

> Sexually transmitted infections (STIs; these include HIV) remain among the greatest infectious disease threats facing the United Kingdom (UK) today. Each year more than 1.5 million new episodes are seen in UK clinics for genitourinary medicine (GUM); and more than 400 000 new STIs are diagnosed in GUM clinics in England alone. Their substantial morbidity, associated mortality, and disproportionate burden on women, marginalised communities, and people with high risk sexual lifestyles continue to drive the prioritisation of STIs in the public health and policy arenas in Britain today. (HPA 2004: 6)

Public concern regarding the increase in the rates of SAI's is reflected in a BBC website on sexual health (BBC 2005). It provides a helpful source of information, using 'pop-up' dialogue boxes with pictures and quotes from young people, practitioners and lay people on their views on sexual health education. The overview of Chlamydia is notable in its representation as a contemporary source of anxiety, signifying a form of sexual 'terrorism' that can be difficult to notice, as often no symptoms are apparent. This 'secret' infection becomes more culturally malign and risky to the individual as infection may result in infertility. Of course, the discursive construction of (sexually acquired) disease as a threat to the culture is not new. Military or wartime metaphors that signify anxiety and danger were particularly visible in relation to HIV/AIDS (Pryce 2005; Sontag 1988). What is particularly apparent in the response and debates around the conduct of sexual activities and health, is the use of language such as 'Defusing the (SAI) time bomb' and the emphasis placed on the individual in the management of their own sexual health.

The statistics around teenage pregnancies and SAIs combine to focus anxiety about young people and the role of education, that tend to polarize around two, familiar, arguments. On the one hand, the increasingly powerful political voice of the 'moral majority' urges a retreat into conventional teaching, espousing sexual abstinence as a means of combating the risk of disease and pregnancy. Once again the risk is configured around knowledge and the value of withholding it as otherwise the individual will discover irresistible, dangerous erotic delights. On the other hand, professional health care practitioners and educators have tended to base the argument on locating the responsibility for assessing and reacting to sexual risk on the individual who should be educated about practices without fear of (too much) moral blame for the erotic activity itself. They do, however run the risk of being blamed for acquiring infection or unintentional pregnancies, especially when they also represent evidence of belonging to socially marginalised or excluded groups, such as migrants, sex workers or the feckless 'Chav' underclass!

The message seems clear for policy makers, health professionals and the individual citizen. The technique of deploying the social regulation of unwanted, negative outcomes of sexual encounters must reside with individual self-surveillance and monitoring; the individual has become the *active patient*, alert to the signs and symptoms of disease and the techniques of risk reduction. In other words, it is no longer taboo to have consensual, legally tolerated sex for pleasure within secular, liberal societies. The responsible citizen is recruited as a medicalised agent of the state, where pleasure is constructed in terms of risk calculation, and 'sin' is predicated on the individual who does not actively employ risk reduction strategies and practices. Of course, this also highlights the quite rapid way that risk is constructed and reconstructed within pathologising discourses. For example, leaflets targeting gay men invite them to join a self-help therapeutic group if they feel 'addicted' to unsafe sex, whereas a decade earlier unsafe sex was 'normal' sex!

The individual – self, risk and sex

As I have already suggested, the individual in any culture must learn 'sexual scripts that are metaphors for conceptualizing the production of behaviour within social life' (Simon 1996: 40). These enable the individual to fulfill the role expected of them, not simply as male or female but also conform to hegemonic notions of sexual performativity or how the person fulfils the social expectations of their gendered/sexual role. In some respects, sexual scripts worked well in relatively stable cultures but are less robust in highly developed and individualistic, rapidly changing societies where the individual may not feel confident with the performance of their 'script'. This a potentially fraught process for most people, for whilst heteronormative rights of passage such as betrothals, marriage and anniversaries are evident in most cultures, they might not represent the 'true' or 'authentic' sexual self of the individual who does not feel part of the dominant sexual order. Rose suggests that psychotherapeutic culture is 'obsessed with the self and how this might be a negative consequence of an earlier (better) state' (1990: 215).

As Plummer (1996) suggests, a rigid and scientific explanation of sex

> is no longer the source of a truth as it was for the moderns with their strong belief in science. Instead, human sexualities became destabilized, decentered and de-essentialised: sexual life is no longer seen as harbouring an essential unitary core locatable within a clear framework (like the nuclear family) with an essential truth waiting to be discovered: there are only fragments. It is ... accompanied by the problematic at every stage. (1996: xiv)

This presents the individual with the most fundamental risk. This risk is that the old narratives that governed what it was to be male or female, in terms of gendered and sexual choreographies and scripts, have been destabilised. Sexual expectations, essentialist assumptions and practices that were familiar to men 40 years ago may now represent anachronistic, sexist views and certainties that some younger men might privately envy and make older men nostalgic for what appear to be more gender determined sexual and social expectations! The process of growing up, the development of sexual maturity and (limited) experimentation with the expectation of 'settling down' in monogamous, heterosexual partnership is no longer necessarily the only socially legitimate path to an 'authentic' sexual identity. However, it is important to remember that such tolerance of diverse identities varies. The individual is engaged in a project that, on the macro level, appears to be reinventing gender such as the 'new man', who is expected to embody the 'civilised', desirable traits of compassion, empathy and increased emotional expression with enhanced sexual performance, erotic sensibilities located within a gym-fit body. Spam e-mails bombard computer users with many entice-ments to increase penis size or sexual performance through tantric exercises or the purchasing of Viagra online. The com-puter is highly accessible and fuels the consumption of arous-ing sexual imagery (which is reputed to be the most common means of transmission of computer viruses) and opportunities for sexually focused interactions with other men and women. In so doing, of course the Internet has become another focus of moral panic, anxiety and a new arena for sexual risk calcu-lation and management.

The rapid development of technologies, social interaction and the challenge to essentialist assumptions of gender are producing new forms of sexual consumption.

As Plummer (1996) elaborates, some of the present trends in sexualities are likely to become increasingly:

Self-conscious and reflective: the very terms we use to discuss sexual-ity will become more discussed, elaborated upon, contexted;

Different in form; from telephone sex to music video erotica, from vir-tual sex to Internet sex cafes;

Differentiated and variable: a plurality of meanings, acts and identities will emerge More recursive, or dependent upon borrowings from the mass media (celebrity cults, soap operas etc) and indeed social sciences;

Indeterminate: a supermarket of sexual possibilities pervades;

Pastiched: these sexual identities blur and change. In the most extreme versions of this story we move beyond human beings and identities'. (1996: xv)

These all represent shifts in the sexual landscape that provide both increased opportunities for sexual pleasure whilst creat-ing new minefields of cultural and biological risk for sexual identities, practices and health. Central in this individualistic consumption is the emphasis on the management of sexual practice that operates within the multi-dimensional opportu-nities and constraints of risk. Once again, male bisexuals are particularly often cited as a risky and largely hidden population who are frequently regarded as a conduit both of disease to their 'innocent' female partners (Gentry and Blair 2003) and distrusted as a subversive threat to 'natural' polarisation of hetero and homosexual orientation. Interestingly, 'girl on girl' bisexual behaviour is often regarded as a particularly pleasurable spectacle for the consumption of heterosexual men!

Managing risk and the venereal threat

The unintended consequences of sexual risk taking tend to be the territory of the health professional – the practitioner as health educator, as well as the politician. For many who identify with the 'moral majority', these diseases or pregnancies signify the dark sin at the heart of religious concerns about sex and the body, which historically locates reproduction rather than recreation as central to discourses around purity and sexual virtue. For many nurses and other health care professionals, sexuality (like gender, class and ethnicity) appears to represent rather risky territory, marginal concerns to be approached with some degree of uncertainty or even embarrassment that must be contained within constantly observed sanitary boundaries of clinical practices. Similarly, considerations of whether the gender or sexual orientation of a patient or client might have any bearing on the social meaning attached to illness and treatments is submerged within the universalising assumptions of the body and disease.

Sex represents powerful symbolic and potentially stigmatising elements in human experience that challenge many of the theoretical and empirically driven frameworks that shape both social and clinical constructions of life. Erotic practices, and the frankly irrational forces of sexual desire that operate in everyday life, have little or no place in the de-sexualized world of the health care arena and clinical practice. In other words, sexuality and medicine are uncomfortable bedfellows, where sex is defined primarily in terms of risks. These risks are located in relation to populations, behaviours and discourses of disease, unwanted pregnancy and non-compliance in treatment regimes.

In addition, sexuality poses a risk to professional health care practice because it may destabilise 'natural' heteronormative categories of 'legitimate' erotic activities and sexual identities. At the heart of practice, is the clinical examination where the performance of controlling the 'erotic charge' demands that the doctor or nurse increase their self-surveillance for signs of their own erotic arousal or transgression of the clinical order. Sexuality is thereby not a condition brought into the clinical arena by the 'other' (patient/client) but is ever present in the interaction, the 'transfer point' of the clinic encounter. As such, the management and control of sexuality and sexual health is not simply located 'out there' but in the conduct of the individual actor – lay or professional.

The dominant medicalised perspectives tend to be focused on epidemiological concerns with the sexual behaviours of specific populations, most notably in relation to the HIV/AIDS pandemic. Following Douglas (1966), it can be seen how as with earlier epidemics of sexually acquired infections (SAI's) such as Syphilis, the public health responses to HIV/AIDS drew on deeply engrained medico-cultural anxieties, taboos and meanings of sin, pollution and the Body. These responses coincided with a heightened public concern of 'green' issues, health and lifestyle and the neo-liberal exhortations to be responsible citizens through emphasis on the body and its governmentality. The re-emergence of syphilis, Chlamydia as well as gonorrhoea and the moral panics around teenage pregnancies, sex work or the legitimisation of gay partnerships (incorrectly depicted as the so-called gay 'marriage') have further emphasised the centrality of 'risk as danger' and the transgressive nature of some sexual categories, identities and behaviours.

Psychosocial theories such as Health Belief Models (Rosenstock 1974) or Rational Choice Theories (Scott 2000) inform some of the somewhat reductive explanations for such apparently risky or socially challenging behaviours. As the theoretical underpinnings of many public health campaigns, such models can be seen to be inconsistent in their effectiveness and might even work to increase resistance to the behavioural changes that are being sought (Coveney and Bunton 2003; Holmes 2005; Lupton 1997). For example, there is an increase in unsafe erotic practice among gay men who prefer unprotected 'bareback' sex despite the lengthy programmes of safer sex education since the emergence of HIV/AIDS pandemic. It is clear that most of these men do understand the potential risk of barebacking yet continue to practice it. In his study of gay men and bathhouses, Holmes (2005) explored the symbolic power of semen exchange as represented by barebacking. 'Barebackers', he argues

> are nomadic subjects (that) reside in the margins of the prescribed 'sexual health': outside the 'acceptable' social norms. They share a common desire: a taste for semen exchange. They induce curiosity, fear and anger because they flirt with danger, contamination, and risk. But they are also, like other marginalized groups, objects of fascination and desire because of their very difference. While semen exchange is commonly viewed as irresponsible and life-threatening, like many other extreme practices (sport, sexual, etc.), it not only inspires 'fear, anxiety and repulsion, but also pleasure, excitement, exhilaration, desire' *Barebackers* are living proof of the dialectic nature of desire and danger. (2005: 19)

In other words both the individuals and their activities represent power, danger and risks that are held in tension through dense networks of sometimes inconsistent erotic and cultural rationalities. Herein, lies the problem for nurses and other health care professionals and educators. A study by Ridge (2004), similarly reveals a celebratory element in the transgressive practice of barebacking but this is also only part of a complex web of contextualised meanings around masculinity and sexual behaviours as well as sensory pleasure. However, whilst barebacking might be mistakenly dismissed by some as having limited appeal outside a specific sexual group, other larger populations may be at risk through underexposure to research and health promotion interventions. Sexual activities must be considered across the lifespan and with changing social structures, the greater flux in the stability of marriage it is clear that older men and women, middle aged bisexuals, the incarcerated (such as prisoners or patients in long stay facilities) also encounter serious biological, social and emotional risk (Farree 2001; Stromberg 2003).

Conclusion

Whilst the traditional concerns of pregnancy and disease remain central to current political and medico-moral discourses around sex, new elements have emerged in the pursuit and consumption of desire and pleasure. These sexual and social practices are, however, also associated with risk discourses and increasing surveillance and deployment of forms of governmentality. One new element is provided by the array of opportunities, technologies for the individual to explore the sometimes surprising or even dangerous boundaries of their erotic potential through the Internet.

The management of social, emotional and intrapsychic risk is also at the heart of new challenges to the conventional categories of sexual identity, through the emergence of categories such as 'metrosexual' or the 'cybersexual'. Like other convenient labels used to signify social types or categories, these represent contemporary aspirations, opportunities and behaviours but also deep tensions between social groups. The 'metrosexual' describes men and women in developed, sophisticated urban environments where sexual behaviours may be highly contextual, and traditional categories (such as orientation) are subverted for example, through bisexuality (Storr 1999). The relative ease with which such behaviours may be adopted by the metrosexual, tend to act as a marker of social status that separate them from social groups who may also be deeply hostile to such challenging threats to traditional beliefs and practices.

The cybersexual, on the other hand, can take this much further and extend post-modern opportunities for pleasure with fewer risks of fumbling over sexual scripts and physical performance through the conduct of 'cybersex', erotic interaction and activities with others or alone. Many heterosexual and non-heterosexual men and women use Internet sex chatrooms to establish relationships and/or explore aspects of desire and sexual expression that hitherto might have been too dangerous to acknowledge, let alone enact in 'real life'. He or she may conduct their sexual activities largely free from the gaze of disapproving neighbours, and are not constrained by the body, class, ethnicity, gender, sexual orientation or adverse biological consequences. The emergence of the cybersexual has further destabilised sexual categories such as 'straight' that have historically been constructed as 'natural' or normal and therefore by definition stand in a binary opposition to the 'other'. The subversion of rigidly maintained gendered and sexual boundaries is sometimes regarded in the popular imagination as troubling and associated with predatory individuals such as paedophiles. However, chat rooms afford the opportunity for men and women to rehearse identities and practices, learning the scripts of other erotic identities that may challenge sexual and gendered performativities whilst retaining anonymity as an element in the calculation of risk. This may be of importance for older men and women who are back, for whatever reason, in the 'dating game'. Many of these people have missed out on safer sex health promotion and are now at 'risk' of infection (Strombeck 2003). There have been incidences of clusters of sexual acquired infections that can be traced back to Internet users who have met up offline. Other risks that have been associated with the use of sex chatrooms include addiction and where numerous cyber (Internet) 'clinics' have been established. These offer therapies along the line of Alcoholics Anonymous and echoing the tendency to construct new medicalising pathologies around sexual practices and pleasure. Many of these Internet sites, particularly those that are US-based, also locate their therapeutic effectiveness within highly moralising 'religious-Right' discourses.

Similarly, the Internet has been exploited by many people to explore and implement sexual desires, but has also been implicated in facilitating adverse biological consequences in particular groups in a post-AIDS environment (Elford *et al.* 2004; Reitmeijer *et al.* 2001). Elford explored how gay men used the Internet to manage sexual encounters but also relationship scripts. His research suggests that the anonymity of the Internet allows HIV positive men to disclose their status more easily than in other settings, for example, bars and clubs, and manage sexual encounters with their concomitant risks.

The resurgence of moral orthodoxies and assertive neo-conservatism are fuelling a backlash against women's rights to calculate risk and manage their own bodies, for instance in relation to birth control, pregnancy and abortion. Similarly, some increasingly confident sexual minorities have become more visible but remain a locus of anxiety and tension, such as the ongoing discord around the appointment of gay priests and bishops. Sadly, such beliefs signify risks to the privileged, 'liberal' assumptions of diversity, as social divisions widen and the anxieties of postmodernity are organised around moral control through the re-assertion of an (illusory) gendered and sexual hegemony based on some notion of a natural order. Despite the apparent relaxing of conventional gendered relations and tolerance of sexual diversity, there remains a dominant normalising element within the social interactions of everyday life. As such, it poses a further challenge to nurses and others who must problematise discriminatory and oppressive assumptions that characterise the taken-for-granted 'natural order' even within the 'rational' order of the clinic.

This chapter has been concerned with risk, sex and most importantly how the individual choreographs his or her erotic career with due attention to the various roles and contexts of everyday life. Inevitably, most of that career constitutes a secret performance around pleasure, desires and the experience of embodiment. There is no doubt that the post-Second World War civil rights and liberation movements, together with the increased visibility of populations organised around sexual identities, have been successful in securing greater legal and social equalities in parts of the world. However, on the other hand, the costs of this focus and acceptance of diverse and insistently vocal and visible sexual discourses remain to be seen. In the meantime, the individual remains thoroughly immersed in navigating his/her way through both the dense interpersonal, social and psychological complexities of erotic desire, and the endless calculations of risk that surround the performance of sexual practices.

11 Final thoughts

Paul Godin

In this book, my fellow contributors and I have applied social theory to provide understanding of how discourse and practices associated with the term risk are relevant to nursing practice. As we have seen, concern about risk within nursing and health care reflects a wider preoccupation with risk in contemporary society (risk society). However, in Chapter 2, Alaszewski makes the point that risk was central to the development and internal structure of health care institutions of the nineteenth century in which modern nursing took shape. Though, as is agued in Chapter 4, it was then understood as 'danger', only later to be understood and managed as 'risk' when institutional confinement gave way to alternative methods of health care. Alaszewski also recognises that changes in the risks health care institutions managed, along with changes in their methods of managing risk, gave rise to community care and modern community nursing. With reference to research data, Alaszewski then points out differences in the ways in which nurses in different areas of community nursing think about and manage risk. Alaszewski's research findings might lead us to ask why, for example, mental health nurses are more inclined to think of risk as a hazard than learning disability nurses, who are more likely to see risk as an opportunity?

The chapters of this book provide something of an answer as to why nurses in particular areas of nursing think of and deal with risk in their own particular ways. In a society in which discourses and practices associated with the term risk have become ever more prevalent they become manifest in nursing in particular ways, depending on the specific field of health care they are related to. As the chapters of this book show, understanding and managing risk involves very different concerns depending on the particular historical development of the area of health care to which it is applied. In Chapter 4 and Chapter 5, we saw how the risk management of mental patients to prevent homicide, violence and suicide has become a major priority for mental health care nurses. Their risk-averse thinking and practices stand in contrast to the risk taking approach of professionals in the field of care for people with learning disabilities, described by Heyman and Davies in Chapter 8. As Heyman and Davies explain, community care of people with learning disability has been led by ideas of normalisation and government policies that emphasise this client group's citizenship and human rights, the exercise of which necessitates active risk taking.

The chapters within the book demonstrate that risk management in nursing in its many forms (care of the unborn child, the child with a life limiting illness, adults defined as having mental illness or learning disabilities and older people) involves conflict between stakeholders (patients, family carers, nurses, other health care workers, the public and policy makers) as they hold opposing views about how risk should be managed, arising from their respective positions, values and interests.

A related theme that might also be gathered from the book is that commonly a trade off exists in managing risk in health care. The prevention of homicide, violence and suicide of mental patients is achieved by restricting their freedom; children with limiting life illnesses could live longer were they to forgo a 'good' childhood; greater safety of people with learning difficulty could be gained at the expense of their autonomy; falls amongst the elderly could be lessened if they led more restricted lifestyles; safe sex involves sacrificing the pleasure and excitement of barebacking. Though this book does not consider all areas of nursing, it should be apparent how this dilemma of risk-averse harm reduction versus risk taking, for the benefits and opportunities the latter affords, cuts across all areas of health care.

As we have seen from this book's various chapters, which choices people make between risk aversion and risk taking, and the many other choices they make regarding risk, are shaped by risk society/reflexive modernity/risk culture/advanced liberalism. As we have seen, Giddens argues that reflexive modernity allows us more informed choice than ever before.

However, even if we accept that this is so, it does not mean that we make independent and fully informed choices about the risks we face. First, our society/culture (be it reflexive modernity or whatever) envelops us, ordering our thinking about risk and the actions we consequently take. Second, as Douglas and Wildavsky (1983) so clearly point out, knowledge about most of the risks we face is infinite and equivocal. The more we know about risks the more we realise the extent of that which we do not of know. Perhaps reflexive modernity makes us less rather than more able to decide on what risks to attend to and how to manage them.

Without the ability to objectively quantify which risks are most and least dangerous (a decision that is itself dependent upon what we value most and least) we are surely free to select which risks we wish to attend to; anything and everything, depending on what we care most and least about. Perhaps with an abundance of knowledge about risks we have just come to worry too much about all the wrong risks. As Tony Blair, the British Prime Minister, asserts 'we are in danger of having a wholly disproportionate attitude to the risks we should expect to run as a normal part of life' (Blair 2005: 1). The prime minister cited as an example:

> one piece of research into a supposed link between autism and the MMR jab, starts a scare that, despite the vast weight of evidence to the contrary, makes people believe a method of vaccination used the world over, is unsafe. (Blair 2005: 1)

He argued that such an attitude and a propensity to regulate for the elimination of risk renders us unable to exploit new scientific discoveries, such that we (in Britain) lose business to India and China. Furthermore, Blair asserted that creativity is stifled in the public sector by this wrong attitude to risk. He thus called for a 'mature' debate about such policies as GM science and for a replacement of 'the compensation culture with a common sense culture' (Blair 2005: 3). Would a mature debate allay the fears Greens have about GM science? Surely whether or not we are in favour of GM farming depends on what we choose to value (economic growth or a safe environment) and what evidence, from an infinite pool of equivocal research findings, we muster to argue that either one is in danger.

Can common sense overcome the propensity to seek compensation as we identify who is to blame? As Douglas asserts, risk is a forensic device. The discourse of risk renders people responsible and accountable for their actions. Thus as Annandale's study (see Chapter 1) and Chapter 3 demonstrate, nurses are continually aware of patients as a source of risk. Patients are seen as ready to accuse and blame nurses for perceived failings in care they receive and/or to be violent towards nurses. How might the application of common sense overcome such a climate of fear? What Dowie (1999), cited in the opening sentences of the introductory chapter, says of the term 'risk' is, perhaps, also true of the term 'common sense', namely that it is a 'conceptual pollutant' that encourages us to assume that we know what we are talking about when we do not. Common sense is assumed to be good sense, though, as Bauman (1997) points out, it has serious limitations. Common sense is based on individuals' limited view of their world and what they regard to be self-evident. Unlike sociology or any other academic discipline, common sense does not subordinate its knowledge to rigorous investigation. Nurses and others might rise to the prime minister's call for: 'a mature, reasoned debate between government, experts and people; a conversation between adults taking responsibility for the risks they face' (Blair 2005). I hope this book proves useful and, more generally, that it helps the reader to get beyond a common sense understanding of risk and nursing practice towards a sociological understanding of risk and nursing practice.

References

Adams J (1995) *Risk*. University College London Press, London.

Adams T (2001) The social construction of risk by community psychiatric nurses and family carers for people with dementia. *Health, Risk & Society*. **3**(3): 307–319.

Alaszewski A (1983) The development of policy for the mentally handicapped since the Second World War. *Oxford Review of Education*. **9**(3): 227–231.

—— (2003) Risk, decision-making and mental health. In Hannigan B and Coffey M (eds) *The Handbook of Community Mental Health Nursing*. Routledge, London. pp. 187–197.

Alaszewski A and Alaszewski H (2002) Towards the creative management of risk: perceptions, practices and policies. *British Journal of Learning Disabilities*. **30**(2): 56–62.

Alaszewski A, Walsh M, Manthorpe J and Harrison L (1997) Managing risk in the city: the role of welfare professionals in managing risks arising from vulnerable individuals in cities. *Health & Place*. **3**(1): 15–23.

Alaszewski A, Alaszewski H, Ayer S and Manthorpe, J. (2000) *Managing Risk in Community Practice: Nursing, Risk and Decision Making*. Balliere Tindall, Edinburgh.

Alaszewski A and Ong B N (eds)(1990) *Normalisation in Practice*. Routledge, London.

Alaszewski A, Harrison L and Manthorpe J (eds)(1998) *Risk, Health and Welfare: Policies, Strategies and Practices*. Open University Press, Buckingham.

Allen D (1979) *Hospital Planning: The Development of the 1962 Hospital Plan: A Case Study in Decision Making*. Pitman Medical, Tunbridge Wells.

Annandale E (1996) Working on the front-line: risk culture and nursing in the new NHS. *Sociological Review*. **44**(3): 416–451.

Anonymous (2004) Verbal abuse of health care staff is a problem we must tackle together. *Nursing Times*. **100**: 31(15), 3rd August.

Armstrong D (1995) The rise of surveillance Medicine. *Sociology of Health & Illness*. **17**(3): 393–404.

Asch D and Hershey J (1995) Why some health policies don't make sense at the bedside. *Annals of Internal Medicine*. **122**(11): 846–850.

Austin J, Oruche U, Dunn D and Levstek D (1995) New-onset childhood seizures: parents' concerns and needs. *Clinical Nursing Practice in Epilepsy.* 2(2): 8–10.

Baker P and Allen D (2001) Physical abuse and physical interventions in learning disabilities: an element of risk? *Journal of Adult Protection.* 3(2): 25–31.

Baldwin S and Thirkettle B (1999) Care in the community for people with a learning disability: choice, opportunity and risk. *Mental Health Care.* 2: 167–169.

Ballinger C and Payne S (2002) The construction of the risk of falling among and by older people. *Ageing and Society.* 22: 305–324.

Barham P (1992) *Closing the Asylum: The Mental Patient in Modern Society.* Penguin, London.

Bath P and Morgan K (1999) Differential risk factor profiles for indoor and outdoor falls in older people living at home in Nottingham, UK. *European Journal of Epidemiology.* 15: 65–73.

Bauman Z (1997) Thinking Sociologically. In Giddens A (ed.) *Sociology: Introductory Readings.* Polity Press, Cambridge, pp. 12–18.

BBC (2005) Sexual Health Website. London: British Broadcasting Corporation. (www.news.bbc.co.uk/1/hi/health/3928539.stm# table Accessed: June 2006)

Beale P (1999) Monitoring violent incidents. In Leather P, Brady C, Lawrence C, Beale P and Cox T (eds) *Work-related Violence: Assessment and Intervention.* Routledge, London, pp. 69–86.

Beck U (1992) *Risk Society: Towards a New Modernity.* Sage, London.

—— (1996) World risk society as cosmopolitan society? Ecological questions in a framework of manufactured uncertainties. *Theory, Culture & Society.* 13(4): 1–32.

Belknap I (1956) *Human Problems of the State Mental Hospital.* McGraw-Hill, New York.

Benner P (1984) *From Novice to Expert: Excellence and Power in Clinical Nursing Practice.* Addison-Wesley, Menlo Park, California.

Bennett G C J and Ebrahim S (1995) *The Esssentials of Health Care in Old Age.*(2nd. edn) Edward Arnold, London.

Bennett D (1991) The international perspective. In Bennett D and Freeman H (eds) *Community Psychiatry: The Principles.* Churchill Livingstone, Edinburgh, pp. 626–649.

Blair A (2005) Speech on Risk and the State. (www.number-10.gov.uk/output/Page7562.asp Accessed: June 2005)

Bodin L, Axelsson G and Ahlborg G (1999) The association of shift work and nitrous oxide exposure in pregnancy with birth weight and gestational age. *Epidemiology.* **10**(4): 429–436.

Bourdieu P (1990) *The Logic of Practice.* Stanford University Press, Stanford.

—— (1995) Social space and symbolic power. In McQuarie, D (ed.) *Readings in Contemporary Sociological Theory: from Modernity to Post-Modernity.* Prentice-Hall, Englewood Cliffs NJ., pp. 323–334.

Bourdieu P and Wacquant L (1992) *An Invitation to Reflexive Sociology.* University of Chicago Press, Chicago.

Brearley C (1982) *Risk and Ageing.* Routledge & Kegan Paul, London.

Bristow J (1997) *Sexuality.* Routledge, London.

Bryan F, Allan T and Russell L (2000) The move from long-stay learning disabilities hospital to community homes: A comparison of clients' nutritional status. *Journal of Human Nutrition & Dietetics.* **13**(4): 365–270.

Budd T (1999) *Violence at Work: Findings from the British Crime Survey.* Home Office, London.

—— (2001) *Violence at Work: New Findings from the 2000 British Crime Survey.* Home Office and Health & Safety Executive, London.

Calgary Health Region (1999) *Preterm Labour.* Previously the Calgary Regional Health Authority, Calgary AB.

—— (2001) *From Here Through Maternity.* Calgary Health Region, Calgary AB.

Campbell M L (1998) Institutional ethnography and experience as data. *Qualitative Sociology.* **21**(1): 55–73.

—— (2001) Textual accounts, ruling action: The intersection of knowledge and power in the routine conduct of community nursing work. *Studies in Cultures, Organizations, and Societies.* **7**(2): 231–250.

Campbell M, Copeland B and Tate B (1998) Taking the standpoint of people with disabilities in research: experiences with participation. *Canadian Journal of Rehabilitation.* **12**(2): 95–104.

Campbell M and Gregor F (2002) *Mapping Social Relations: A Primer in Doing Institutional Ethnography.* Garamond Press, Aurora, ON.

Cambridge P (2004) Abuse inquiries as learning tools for social care organisations. In Stanley N and Manthorpe J (eds) *The Age of Inquiry: Learning and Blaming in Health and Social Care.* Routledge, London, pp. 231–254.

Canadian Perinatal Surveillance System(CPSS) (2003) *Canadian Perinatal Health Report.* Health Canada, Ottawa.

Caplan P (1998) Mother-blaming. In Ladd-Taylor M and UmanskyL (eds) *'Bad' Mothers: The Politics of Blame in Twentieth Century America.* New York University Press, New York, pp. 127–144.

Caplan G (1964) *Principles of Preventive Psychiatry.* Basic Books, New York.

Carlton-Ford S, Miller R, Nealeigh N and Sanchez N (1997) The effects of perceived stigma and psychological over-control on the behavioural problems of children with epilepsy. *Seizure.* 6(5): 383–391.

Carnard G (1996) Falling trend. *Nursing Times.* 92(1): 36–38.

Carter S, Campbell E, Sanson-Fisher R, Redman S and Gillespie W (1997) Environmental hazards in the homes of older people. *Age and Ageing.* 26(3): 195–202.

Castel R (1988) *The Regulation of Madness.* Polity Press, Cambridge.

—— (1991) From dangerousness to risk. In Burchell G, Gordon C and Miller P (eds) *The Foucault Effect: Studies in Governmentality.* Harvester Wheatsheaf, London, pp. 281–298.

Cembrowicz S P and Shepherd J P (1992) Violence in the accident and emergency department. *Medicine, Science and the Law.* 32(2): 118–122.

Chambers E and Oakhill A (1995) Models of care for children dying of cancer. *Palliative Medicine.* 9(3): 181–185.

Chappell A L (1994) A question of friendship: community care and the relationships of people with learning difficulties. *Disability and Society.* 9(4): 419–433.

Clemson L, Cusick A and Fozzards C (1999) Managing risk and exerting control: determining follow through with falls prevention. *Disability and Rehabilitation.* 21(12): 531–541.

Cockerham W, Rutten A and Abel T (1997) Conceptualizing contemporary health lifestyles: moving beyond Weber. *Sociological Quarterly.* 38(2): 321–342.

Committee of Public Accounts, H. o. C. (2003) *Protecting NHS Hospital and Ambulance Staff from Violence and Aggression: 39th Report, Session 2002–3.* Stationery Office, London.

Constantinos P (2003) Greek Sexual Culture, Identity and Ethnicity. (www.lse.ac.uk/collections/hellenicObservatory/pdf/symposiumPapersonline/Phellas.pdf Accessed: June 2005)

Coombes R (1999) Why are nurses more at risk than these bouncers? *Nursing Times.* 95: 17.

Cooper H (2002) Investigating socio-economic explanations for gender and ethnic inequalities in health. *Social Science & Medicine.* 54(5): 693–706.

Corkish C and Heyman B (1998) The resettlement of people with severe learning difficulties. In Heyman B (ed.) *Risk, Health and Health Care: A Qualitative Approach.* Edward Arnold, London, pp. 215–227.

Coveney J and Bunton R (2003) In pursuit of the study of pleasure: implications for health research and practice. *Health: An Interdisciplinary Journal for the Social Study of Health, Illness and Medicine.* 7(2): 161–179.

Coyle D and Northway R (1999) Promoting health: the challenge for the community learning disability nurse. *Mental Health Care.* 2(7): 232–235.

Crowner, M L, Peric, G, Stepcic, F and Van Oss, E (1994) A comparison of videocameras and official incident reports in detecting inpatient assaults. *Hospital and Community Psychiatry.* 45(11): 1144–1145.

Darling R (1979) *Families Against Society: A Study of Reactions to Children with Birth Defects.* Sage, London.

Daviss B (1997) Heeding warnings from the canary, the whale, and the Inuit. In Davis-Floyd R and Sargent C (eds) *Childbirth and Authoritative Knowledge.* University of California Press, Berkeley, pp. 441–473.

Dean M (1997) Sociology after society. In Owen D(ed.) *Sociology after Postmodernism.* Sage, London, pp. 205–228.

Denscombe M (1993) Personal Health and the social psychology of risk taking. *Health Education Research.* 8(4): 505–517.

Department of Health (1989) *Caring for people.* HMSO, London.

—— (1990) *NHS & Community Care Act.* HMSO, London.

—— (1992) *The Health of the Nation: A Strategy for Health in England.* HMSO, London.

—— (1995) *Mental Health (Patients in the Community) Act 1995: Chapter 52,* HMSO, London.

—— (1999a) *Saving Lives: Our Healthier Nation.* The Stationery Office, London.

—— (1999b) *Health Service Circular 99/226. Campaign to stop violence against staff working in the NHS: NHS Zero Tolerance Zone.* Department of Health, London.

—— (1999c) *We Don't Have to Take This: Resource Pack.* NHS Executive, Leeds.

—— (1999d) *Working Together – securing a quality workforce for the NHS: Health Service Circular 1999/079 and 1999/229.* Department of Health, London.

—— (2000a) *Building a Safer NHS for Patients: Implementing an Organisation with a Memory.* The Stationery Office, London.

—— (2000b) *Improving Working Lives.* Department of Health, London.

—— (2000c) *NHS Day Care Facilities England Financial Year 1999–00.* Department of Health, London.

—— (2001a) *National Service Framework for Older People.* The Stationery Office, London.

—— (2001b) *Care Homes for Older People: National Minimum Standards.* The Stationery Office, London.

—— (2002) *National Strategy for Sexual Health & HIV: Implementation Action Plan.* (www.doh.gov.uk/sexualhealthandhiv Accessed: June 2005)

—— (2004) *Choosing Health: Making Healthier Choices Easier.* The Stationery Office, London.

—— (2004b) *Improving Mental Health Law – Towards a new Mental Health Act,* The Stationery Office, London.

—— (2004c) *Choosing Health? A consultation on improving people's health.* (www.dh.gov.uk/Consultations/ClosedConsultations/ClosedConsultationsArticle/fs/en?CONTENT_ID=4084418&chk=u9aLWB Accessed: June 2005)

—— (2005) Chief Nursing Officer demands Action for Cleaner, Safer Hospitals. (www.dh.gov.uk/PublicationsAndStatistics/PressReleases/PressReleasesNotices/fs/en?CONTENT_ID=4104425&chk=LSeM2O. Accessed: February 2005)

Department of Health and Human Services (2001) The Surgeon General's Call To Action To Promote Sexual Health And Responsible Sexual Behavior. (www.surgeongeneral.gov/library/sexualhealth/call.htm Accessed: June 2005)

DeVault M L and McCoy L (2002) Institutional ethnography: Using interviews to investigate ruling relations. In Gubrium J F and Holstein J A (eds) *Handbook of Interview Research: Context and Method,* Sage Publications, Thousand Oaks, pp. 751–776.

Dewing J (1999) Dementia part 4: risk management. *Professional Nurse.* **14**(11): 803–805.

Diamond T (1992) *Making Gray Gold: Narratives of Nursing Home Care.* University of Chicago Press, Chicago.

Douglas M (1966) *Purity and Danger: Conceptions of Pollution and Taboos.* Routledge and Kegan Paul, London.

—— (1986) *How Institutions Think.* Syracuse University Press, New York.

—— (1986) *Risk Acceptability According to the Social Sciences.* Routledge and Kegan Paul, London.

—— (1990) Risk as a forensic resource, Daedalus. *Journal of the American Academy of Arts and Sciences.* **119**(4): 1–6.

Douglas M (1992) *Risk and Blame: Essays in Cultural Theory.* Routledge, London.

Douglas M and Wildavsky A (1983) *Risk and culture: An Essay on the Selection of Technological and Environmental Dangers.* University of California Press, London.

Dowie J (1999) Communication for better decisions: not about risk. *Health, Risk & Society.* 1(1): 41–53.

Dowswell T, Towner E, Cryer C, Jarvis S, Edwards P and Lowe P (1999) *Accidental Falls: Fatalities and Injuries: An Examination of the Data Sources and Review of the Literature on Preventive Strategies.* A Report prepared for the Department of Trade and Industry, University of Newcastle and South East Institute of Public Health, University of London, London.

Eayrs C B, Ellis N and Jones R S P (1993) Which label? An investigation into the effects of terminology on public perceptions of and attitudes towards people with learning difficulties. *Disability, Handicap & Society.* 8(2): 111–127.

Edwardson S (1983) The choice between hospital and home care for terminally ill children. *Nursing Research.* 32(1): 29–34.

Eiser C, Haverman T, Pancer M and Eiser J (1992) Adjustment to chronic disease in relation to age and gender: mother's and father's reports of their children's behaviour. *Journal of Pediatric Psychology.* 17(3): 261–275.

Eldridge J and Hill A (1999) Thinking about risk: a review essay. *Health, Risk and Society.* 1(3): 343–350.

Elford J, Bolding G, Davis M, Sherr L and Hart G (2004) web-based behavioral surveillance among men who have sex with men: a comparison of online and offline samples in London, UK. *JAIDS Journal of Acquired Immune Deficiency Syndromes.* 35(4): 421–426.

Elston M A, Gabe J, Denney D, Lee R and O'Beirne M. (2002) Violence against doctors: a medical(ised) problem? The case of National Health Service general practitioners, *Sociology of Health and Illness.* 24(5): 575–598.

Emond A and Eaton N (2004) Supporting children with complex health care needs and their families – an overview of the research agenda. Child: Care. *Health & Development* 30(3): 195–199.

Enkin M and Keirse M (2000) *A Guide to Effective Care in Pregnancy and Childbirth* (3rd edn) Oxford University Press, Toronto.

Esterberg K G (2002) The bisexual menace: Or, will the real bisexual stand up? In Richardson D and Seidman S (eds) *Handbook of Lesbian and Gay Studies.* Sage, London, pp. 215–227.

Esterberg L, Horton K, Arber S and Davidson K (2001) *International Review of Interventions in Falls among Older People.* Department of Trade and Industry/Health development Agency.

Farrell G A (2001) From tall poppies to squashed weeds: why don't nurses pull together more? *Journal of Advanced Nursing.* **35**(1): 26–33.

Faubion J D (1993) *Modern Greek Lessons: A Primer in Historical Constructivism.* Princeton University Press, New Jersey.

Ferguson P (2001) Mapping the family: disability studies and the exploration of parental responses to disability. In G Albrecht, G, Seelman, K and Bury, M (eds) *Handbook of Disability Studies.* Sage, London, pp. 373–395.

Ferree M C (2001) Females and sex addiction: Myths and diagnostic Implications. *Sexual Addiction & Compulsivity.* **8**(3): 287–300.

Flynn R (2002) Clinical goverance and governmentality. *Health, Risk & Society.* **4**(2): 155–173.

Foucault M (1971) *Madness & Civilization: A History in the Age of Reason.* Social Science Paperback, Tavistock Publications, London.

—— (1978) *The History of Sexuality Vol. 1.* Penguin, London.

—— (1979) *Discipline and Punish: The Birth of the Prison.* Penguin, Harmondsworth.

—— (1980) *Power/Knowledge: Selected Interviews and Other Writings 1972–1977. Edited by Colin Gordon.* Pantheon, New York.

—— (1989) *Foucault Live (Interviews 1966–84).* Semiotext, Columbia University, New York.

—— (1991) Governmentality. In Burchell G, Gordon C and Miller P (eds) *The Foucault Effect: Studies in Governmentality.* Harvester Wheatsheaf, London. pp. 87–104.

Fox N (1995) Postmodern perspectives on care: the vigil and the gift. *Critical Social Policy* **15**(4): 107–125.

—— (1998) 'Risks', 'Hazards' and life choices: reflections on health at work. *Sociology.* **32**(4): 665–687.

Freidson E (1970) *Profession of Medicine, a Study of the Sociology of Applied Knowledge.* Harper Row, New York.

French G (2005) Speech Summary. (www.dh.gov.uk/NewsHome/ ConferenceAndEventReports/ConferenceReportsConferenceRep ortsArticle/fs/en?CONTENT_ID=4102049&chk=GgHAEH. Accessed: February 2005)

Freshwater D (2000) Crosscurrents: against cultural narration in nursing. *Journal of Advanced Nursing.* **32**(2): 481–484.

Furedi F (2001) *Paranoid Parenting: Abandon your Anxieties and be a Good Parent.* Allen Lane and Penguin, London.

Gabriel A and Bowling A (2004) Quality of Life from the perspectives of older people. *Ageing and Society.* **24**(5): 675–691.

Gentry A C and Blair J M (2003) The extent of bisexual behaviour in HIV infected men and implications for transmission to their female sex partners. *AIDS Care.* **15**(6): 829–837.

Gami A (2002) Sexual Health: The emergence, development, and diversity of a Concept. *Annual Review of Sex Research.* **X111**: 1–35.

Giddens A (1990) *The Consequences of Modernity.* Polity Press, Cambridge.

—— (1991) *Modernity and Self-Identity: Self and Society in the late Modern Age.* Polity Press, Cambridge.

—— (1992) *The Transformation of Intimacy: Sexuality, Love & Eroticism in Modernism.* Polity, Oxford.

—— (1994) Agenda change. *New Society and Statesman.* 7(323) (October): 23–25.

—— (1998) *The Third Way: The Renewal of Social Democracy.* Polity Press, Cambridge.

Gliedman J and Roth W (1980) *The Unexpected Minority: Handicapped Children in America.* Harcourt Brace Jovanovitch, New York.

Godin P (2004) 'You don't tick boxes on a form': A study of how community mental health nurses assess and manage risk. *Health, Risk & Society.* **6**(4): 347–360.

Goffman E (1961) *Asylums: Essays on the Social Situation of Mental Patients and Other Inmates.* Pelican Books, Harmonsworth.

—— (1970) *Stigma: Notes on the Management of Spoilt Identity.* Penguin, Harmondsworth.

Goldenberg R L and Rouse D J (1998) Prevention of premature birth. *The New England Journal of Medicine.* **339**(5): 313–320.

Goodman C, Woolley R and Knight D (2003) District nurses' experiences of providing care in residential care home settings. *Journal of Clinical Nursing.* **12**(1): 67–76.

Goodwin S (1997) *Comparative Mental Health Policy: From Institutional to Community Care.* Sage, London.

Gosselin C, Robitailee Y, Trickey F and Maltias D (1993) Factors predicting the implementation of home modifications among elderly people with loss of independence. *Physical and Occupational Therapy in Geriatrics.* **12**(1): 15–23.

Gould J (2004) Press Release on Independent Advisory Group (www.dh.gov.uk/assetRoot/04/08/41/67/04084167.doc Accessed: June 2005)

Gould M (2004) Report accuses NHS of institutional racism. *British Medical Journal.* **328**: 367.

Gournay K (2002) *The Recognition, Prevention and Therapeutic Management of Violence in Mental Health Care. A Consultation Document prepared for the United Kingdom Central Council for Nursing, Midwifery and Health Visiting.* UKCC, London.

Government of Alberta, Human Resources and Employment (2004) Becoming a Parent in Alberta: What you Need to Know About Human Rights, Maternity and Parental leave, and Benefits. (www.albertahumanrights.ab.ca/publications/Becoming a Parent/index.asp. Accessed: June 2005)

Green S (2003) "What do you mean 'what's wrong with ?' ": Stigma and the lives of families of children with disabilities. *Social Science & Medicine.* **57**(8): 1361–1374.

Grinyer A (1995) Risk, the real world and naive sociology: perceptions of risk from occupational injury in the health service. In Gabe J (ed.) *Medicine, Health and Risk: Sociological Approaches.* Blackwell Science, Oxford, pp. 31–51.

Harding J (1997) Bodies at risk: sex, surveillance and hormone replacement therapy. In Petersen A and Bunton R (eds) *Foucault, Health and Medicine.* Routledge, London, pp. 134–150.

Hart C (2004) *Nurses and Politics: The Impact of Power and Practice.* Macmillan, Basingstoke.

Hays S (1996) *The Cultural Contradictions of Motherhood.* Yale University Press, New Haven, CT.

Health Services Advisory Committee (1997) *Violence and Aggression to Staff in the Health Services.* Health and Safety Executive, London.

Healthcare Commission (2004) *2003* NHS Staff Survey. (www.healthcarecommission.org.uk/staffsurveys Accessed: March 2005)

—— (2005) NHS Staff Survey 2004. (www.healthcarecommission.org.uk/staffsurveys Accessed: March 2005)

Health Protection Agency (2004) Focus on Prevention: HIV and other Sexually Transmitted Infections in the United Kingdom in 2003. Annual Report. (www.hpa.org.uk/infections/topics_az/hiv_and_sti/publications/annual2004/annual2004.htm Accessed: June 2005)

Heaman M I, Sprague A E and Stewart P J (2001) Reducing the preterm birth rate: A population health strategy. *Journal of Obstetric, Gynecologic, and Neonatal Nursing.* **30**(1): 20–29.

Hearn J and Parkin W (2001) *Gender, Sexuality and Violence in Organizations: The Unspoken Forces of Organization Violations.* Sage, London and Thousand Oaks, CA.

Heiman T (2002) Parents of children with disabilities: resilience, coping and future expectations. *Journal of Developmental and Physical Disabilities.* **14**(2): 159–171.

Hensyl W R (ed) (1990) *Stedman's medical dictionary. (25th ed.).* Williams & Wilkins, Baltimore MD.

Heyman B and Huckle S (1993a) Not worth the risk? Attitudes of adults with learning difficulties and their informal and formal carers to the hazards of everyday life. *Social Science & Medicine.* 12(37): 1557–1564.

——— (1993b) Normal life in a hazardous world: How adults with moderate learning difficulties and their carers cope with risks and dangers. *Disability, Handicap & Society.* 8(2): 143–160.

——— (1995) How adults with learning difficulties and their carers see 'the community'. In Heyman B (ed.) *Researching User Perspectives on Community Health Care.* Chapman Hall, London, pp. 165–182.

Heyman B, Swain J Gillman M, Handyside E C and Newman W (1997) Alone in the crowd: How adults with learning difficulties cope with social network problems. *Social Science & Medicine.* 44(2): 41–53.

Heyman B, Huckle S and Handyside E C (1998) Freedom of the locality for people with learning difficulties. In Heyman B (ed.) *Risk, Health and Health Care: A Qualitative Approach.* Edward Arnold, London, pp.199–214.

Heyman B, Swain J and Gillman M (2004) Organisational simplification and secondary complexity in health services for adults with learning disabilities. *Social Science & Medicine.* 58(2): 357–367.

Heyman B, Shaw M, Davies J, Godin P, and Reynolds L (2004) Forensic mental health services as a risk escalator: a case study in ideals and practice. *Health, Risk and Society.* 6(4): 307– 325.

Higgs P (1998) Risk, governmentality and the reconceptualisation of citizenship. In Scambler G and Higgs P (eds) *Modernity, Medicine and Health: Medical Sociology towards 2000.* Routledge, London, pp. 176–197.

Hirsch J (1991) Fordism and Post-Fordism. In Bonefeld W and Holloway J (eds) *Post-Fordism and Social Form a Marxist Debate on the Post-Fordist State.* Macmillan. London, pp. 8–34.

Holmes D (2005) The anatomy of a forbidden desire: men, penetration and semen exchange. *Nursing Inquiry.* 12(1): 10–19.

Home Office and Department of Health & Social Security (1975) *Report of the Committee on Mentally Abnormal Offenders.* (Butler Report) HMSO, London.

Horton K (2002) *Gender and Falls: Perceptions of Older People and their Family Members.* Unpublished PhD thesis. University of Surrey.

Horton K and Arber S (2004) Gender and the negotiation between older people and their carers in the prevention of falls. *Ageing and Society.* 23(1): 75–94.

Hughes M (2002) Fall prevention and the national service framework. *Nursing Standard.* 17(4): 33–38.

International Labour Organisation, International Council of Nurses, World Health Organisation, & Public Services International (2002) *Framework Guidelines for Addressing Workplace Guidelines in the Health Sector.* Geneva.

James A (2000) Embodied being(s): understanding the self and he body in childhood. In A Prout (ed.) *The Body, Childhood and Society.* Macmillan. London, pp.19–37.

Jay P (1979) *Report of the Committee of Enquiry into Mental Handicap Nursing and Care.* HMSO, London.

Jenkins R (2002) Learning disability nursing. Value of employment to people with learning disabilities. *British Journal of Nursing.* 11(1): 38–45.

Jensen J, Nyberg L, Gustafson Y and Lundin-Olsson L (2003) Fall and injury prevention in residential care- effects in residents with higher and lower levels of cognition. *Journal of American Geriatrics Society.* 51(5): 627–635.

Kelley P, Mayall B and Hood S (1997) Children's accounts of risk. *Childhood* 4(3): 305–324.

Kelly L and Radford J (1996) 'Nothing really happened': the invalidation of women's experience of sexual violence. In Hester M, Kelly L and Radford J (eds) *Women, Violence and Male Power.* Open University Press, Buckingham, pp.19–33.

Kelly L S and McKenna H P (1997) Victimisation of people with enduring mental illness in the community. *Journal of Psychiatric and Mental Health Nursing.* 4(3): 185–191.

Kemshall H (1998) *Risk in Probation Practice.* Ashgate, Aldershot.

—— (2000) Conflicting knowledges on risk: the case of risk knowledge in the probation service. *Health, Risk and Society.* 2(2): 143–158.

—— (2002) *Risk, Social Policy and Welfare.* Open University Press, Buckingham.

Kerr M, Fraser W and Felce D (1996) Primary health care for people with a learning disability: A keynote review. *British Journal of Learning Disabilities.* 24(1): 2–8.

Kevles D (1985) *In the Name of Eugenics.* University of California Press, Berkley.

Kingston P (1998) *Older People and Falls: A Randomised Control Trial on Health Visitor Intervention.* Unpublished Ph D thesis. Keele University.

Kirk S and Glendinning C (2004) Developing services to support parents caring for a technology-dependent child at home. *Child: Care, Health & Development.* 30 (3): 209–218.

Kramer M S, Seguin L, Lydon J and Goulet L (2000) Socio-economic disparities in pregnancy outcome: why do the poor fare so poorly? *Paediatric and Perinatal Epidemiology.* 14(3): 194–210.

Kunkler I (2000) Managed clinical networks: a new paradigm for clinical medicine. *Journal of the Royal College of Physicians.* 34(3): 230–233.

Lahire B (2003) From the habitus to an individual heritage of dispositions. Towards a sociology at the level of the individual. *Poetics.* 31(5): 329–355.

Lam A (2000) Tacit knowledge, organizational learning and societal institutions—an integrated framework. *Organizational Studies.* 21(3): 487–513.

Landsman G (2003) Emplotting children's lives: developmental delay vs. disability. *Social Science & Medicine.* 56(9): 1947–1960.

Larson E (1998) Reframing the meaning of disability to families: the embrace of paradox. *Social Science & Medicine.* 47(7): 865–875.

Lash S (1992) Reflexive modernization: the aesthetic dimension. *Theory, Culture & Society.* 10(3) 1–23.

—— (2000) Risk culture. In Adams B, Beck U and Van Loon J (eds)*The Risk Society and Beyond.* Sage, London, pp. 47–62.

Lawler J (1991) *Behind the Screens Nursing, Somology, and the Problem of the Body.* Churchill Livingstone, Edinburgh.

Lawton M P, Moss M and Dunamel L M (1995) The quality of life among elderly care receivers. *Journal of Applied Gerontology.* 14(2): 150–171.

Lee R M (1995) *Dangerous Fieldwork.* Sage, London and Thousand Oaks.

Lee R M and Stanko E A(eds) (2003) *Researching Violence: Essays on Methodology and Measurement.* Routledge, London.

Lemke T (2001) 'The birth of bio-politics': Michel Foucault's lecture at the Collège de France on neo-liberal governmentality, *Economy and Society.* 30(2): 190–207.

Lenton S, Stallard P, Lewis M and Mastroyannopoulou K (2001) Prevalence and morbidity associated with non-malignant, life-threatening conditions in childhood. *Child: Care, Health & Development* 27(5): 389–398.

Lipsky M (1980) *Street-level Bureaucracy: Dilemmas of the Individual in Public Services.* Russell Sage Foundation, New York.

Lloyd L (2004) Mortality and Morality: ageing and the ethics of care. *Ageing and Society.* 24(2): 235–256.

Lomax M (1921) *The Experiences of an Asylum Doctor: With Suggestions for Asylum and Lunacy Law Reform.* George Allen & Unwin, London.

Lord S R, Sherrington C and Menz H (2001) *Falls in Older people: Risk Factors and Strategies for Prevention.* Cambridge University Press, Cambridge.

Lumley J (2003) Defining the problem: the epidemiology of preterm birth. *BJOG: an International Journal of Obstetrics and Gynaecology.* **110** (Supplement 20): 3–7.

Lupton D (1995) *The Imperative of Health: Public Health and the Regulated Body.* Sage, London.

—— (1997) *The Imperative of Health: Public Health and the Regulated Body.* Sage, Thousand Oaks.

—— (1999) *Risk.* Routledge, London.

Ly L and Howard D (2004) *Statistics of mentally disordered offenders 2003: England and Wales.* Home Office Statistical Bulletin 16/04, Home Office, London.

Lyotard J F (1979) *La condition postmoderne: rapport sur le savoir.* Cited in Turner (1993) Regulating Bodies. Routledge, London.

MacDonald C, Redondo V, Baetz R and Boyle M (1993) Obstetrical triage. *The Canadian Nurse.* **89**(7)(August): 17–20.

Manthorpe J (2001) Managing risk in learning disabilities services: Issues emerging from the new learning disabilities strategy. *Managing Community Care.* **9**(1): 42–47.

Manthorpe J, and Alaszewski A (2000) Service users, informal carers and risk. In Alaszewski A, Harrision L and Manthorpe J (eds) *Risk, Health and Welfare.* Open University Press, Buckingham, pp. 47–70.

Marcoulatos J (2001) Merleau-Ponty and Bourdieu on embodied significance. *Journal for the Theory of Social Behaviour.* **31**(1): 1–27.

Martinson I, Moldow D and Armstrong G (1986) Home care for children dying of cancer. *Research in Nursing & Health.* **9**(1): 11–16.

Masterson A (1999) Nursing older people in hospital. In Redfern S and Ross F (eds) *Nursing Older People.* (3rd edn) Churchill Livingstone, London, pp. 123–139.

McCoy L (in press) Keeping the institution in view: Working with interview accounts of everyday experience. In Smith D E (ed.) *Institutional Ethnography as Practice.* AltaMira, Walnut Creek.

McKeever P and Miller K-L (2004) Mothering children who have disabilities: a Bourdieusian interpretation of maternal practices. *Social Science & Medicine.* **59**(6): 1177–1191.

McKeown T (1979) *The Role of Medicine: Dream, Mirage or Nemesis?* (2nd edn) Blackwell, Oxford.

Meisenhelder T (1997) Pierre Bourdieu and the call for a reflexive sociology. *Current Perspectives in Social Theory* **17**: 159–183.

Messent P R, Cooke C B and Long J (1999) Primary and secondary barriers to physically healthy lifestyles foe adults with learning disabilities. *Disability & Rehabilitation.* **21**(9): 409–419.

Mest G M (1988) With a little help from their friends: Use of social support systems by persons with retardation. *Journal of Social Issues.* **44**(1): 117–125.

Miesen B (1995) Awareness in Alzheimer's disease patients: consequences for caregiving research. Paper presented at III European Congress of Gerontology, 30th August-2nd September, 1995.

Minichiello V, Browne J and Kendig H (2000) Perceptions and consequences of ageism: views of older people. *Ageing and Society.* **20**(3): 253–278.

Ministry of Health (1962) *Hospital Plan for England and Wales, Cmd 1604.* HMSO, London.

Ministry of Health (1963) *Health and Welfare Plan, Cmd 1963.* HMSO, London.

Morgan H (2003) Count us: The inquiry into meeting the mental health needs of young people with learning disabilities. *Tizard Learning Disability Review.* **8**(3): 37–43.

Moss N E (2002) Gender equity and socioeconomic inequality: a framework for the patterning of women's health. *Social Science & Medicine.* **54**(5): 649–661.

Moutquin J M (2003) Socio-economic and psychosocial factors in the management and prevention of preterm labour. *BJOG: an International Journal of Obstetrics & Gynaecology.* **110** (Supplement 20): 56–60.

Mozurkewich E L, Luke B, Avni M and Wolf F M (2000) Working conditions and adverse pregnancy outcome: A meta-analysis. *Obstetrics & Gynecology.* **95**(4): 623–635.

Murphy E (2000) Risk, responsibility, and rhetoric in infant feeding. *Journal of Contemporary Ethnography.* **29**(3): 291–325.

Mykhalovskiy E (2001) Troubled hearts, care pathways and hospital restructuring: Exploring health services research as active knowledge. *Studies in Cultures, Organizations, and Societies.* **7**(2): 269–296.

Mykhalovskiy E and McCoy L (2002) Troubling ruling discourses of health: Using institutional ethnography in community-based research. *Critical Public Health.* **12**: 17–37.

National Audit Office (2003a) *A Safer Place to Work: Improving the management of health and safety risks to staff in NHS Trusts: Report by the Comptroller and Auditor General.* Stationery Office, London.

—— (2003b) *A Safer Place to Work: Protecting NHS Hospital and Ambulance Staff from Violence and Aggression: Report by the Comptroller and Auditor General.* Stationery Office, London.

National Institute for Clinical Excellence (NICE) (2005) *Violence: the Short-term Management of Disturbed/Violent Behaviour in Psychiatric In-patient Settings and Emergency Departments.* (www.nice.org.uk 26/02/05. Accessed: March 2005)

Narayan S M and Corcoran-Perry S (1997) Lines of reasoning as a representation of nurses' clinical decision making. *Research in Nursing and Health.* **20**(4): 353–364.

Needham I, Abderhalden C, Halfens R J G, Fischer, J E and Dassen T (2005) Non-somatic effects of patient aggression on nurses: a systematic review. *Journal of Advanced Nursing.* **49**(3): 283–296.

Nettleton S (1997) Governing the risky self: how to become healthy, wealthy and wise. In Petersen A and Bunton R (eds) *Foucault, Health and Medicine.* Routledge, London, pp. 207–222.

Neysmith S M (2000) Networking across difference: Connecting restructuring and caring labour. In Neysmith S M (ed.) *Restructuring Caring Labour: Discourse, State Practice, and Everyday Life.* Oxford University Press, Toronto, pp. 1–28.

NHS Executive (2001a) *NHS Zero Tolerance Zone Campaign: Phase III.* NHS Executive, Leeds.

—— (2001b) *Zero Tolerance Zone Phase IV:Withholding Treatment from Violent and Abusive Patients in NHS Trusts.* NHS Executive, Leeds. HSC 2001/18.

—— (2002) *Dealing with Harassment by NHS Service Users- A guide for managers and staff.* NHS Executive, Leeds.

—— (2003) *NHS Zero Tolerance Zone. Campaign Update 31-7-03.*

Niday P and Kinch R (1998) *Preterm Birth Consensus Conference: Report and Background Papers.* 24th to 25th April 1998, Ottawa.

Noble P and Rodger S (1989) Violence by psychiatric in-patients. *British Journal of Psychiatry.* **155**: 384–390.

Norris, R. (2004) The shocking truth about verbal abuse. *Nursing Times.* **100**(31)(3 August): 12–13.

Nursing and Midwifery Council(NMC) (2004) *The Management of Violence-Changing a Culture.* (www.nmc-uk.org/nmc Accessed: Ocober 2004)

—— (2004a) *Risk Management.* (www.nmc-uk.org/nmc/main/advice/riskManagement.html: Accessed: June 2005)

—— (2004b) *Clinical Governance.* (www.nmc-uk.org/nmc/main/advice/clinicalGovernance.html: Accessed: June 2005)

Nyberg L and Gustafson Y (1995) Patient falls in stroke rehabilitation: A challenge to rehabilitation strategies. *Stroke.* **26**(5): 838–842.

Oliver D, Britton M and Seed P (1997) Development and evaluation of evidence-based risk assessment tool (STRATIFY) to predict which elderly inpatients will fall. *British Medical Journal.* **315**(7115): 1049–1053.

Oliver M (1990) *The Politics of Disability.* Macmillan, Basingstoke.

Osborne T (1993) On liberalism, neo-liberalism and the 'liberal profession' of Medicine. *Economy and Society.* **22**(3): 345–356.

Oxtoby K (2004) Silence the abuse. *Nursing Times.* **100**(31) (31 August): 22–25. Papiernik E (1999) Fetal growth retardation: A limit for the further reduction of preterm births. *Maternal and Child Health Journal.* **3**(2): 63–69.

Parrish A and Styring L (2003) Learning disability nursing. Nurses' role in the developments in learning disability care. *British Journal of Nursing.* **12**(17): 1043–1047.

Parse R (1987) *Nursing Science: Major Paradigms, Theories and Critiques.* W.B. Saunders, Philadelphia.

Paterson B and Leadbetter D (1999) Managing physical violence. In Turnball J and Paterson B (eds). *Aggression and Violence.* Macmillan, Basingstoke, pp. 124–127.

Petersen A (1997) Risk, governance and the new public health. In Petersen A and Bunton R (eds) *Foucault, Health and Medicine.* Routledge, London, pp. 189–205.

Phillip M and Duckworth D (1982) *Children with Disabilities and Their Families: A Review Of Research.* NFER-Nelson Publishing, Berkshire.

Pickering S and Thompson JS (eds) *Promoting Positive Practice in Nursing Older People.* Bailliere Tindall, London.

Pickett K E (1999) *Social Context, Race/Ethnicity and Preterm Birth.* (Doctoral Dissertation, University of California, Berkeley), Retrieved July 15, 2004 from UMI ProQuest Digital Dissertations (UMI Number: 9931364).

Plummer K (1996) Foreward. In Simon W (1996) *Postmodern Sexualities.* Routledge, London, pp. ix–xvi.

Porter E J (1994) Older widows' lived experience of 'risk': how they articulated the risks they experienced and ways in which they attempted to reduce these risks. *Advances in Nursing Science.* **17**(2): 54–65.

Poster E and Ryan J (1993) At risk of assault. *Nursing Times.* **89**: 30–33.

RIDDOR (Reporting of Injuries, Diseases and Dangerous Occurrences Regulations). (1995) HMSO, London.

Procter S (2002) Whose evidence? Agenda setting in multi-professional research:observations from a case-study. *Health, Risk and Society.* **4**(1): 43–59.

Prout A (2000) Childhood bodies: social construction and translation. In Williams S, Gabe J and Calnan M (eds) *Health, Medicine And Society: Key Theories, Future Agendas.* Routledge, London, pp.109–122.

Pryce A (2000) 'Does your mother know you are heterosexual?': Discretion management and resistance of the erotic in the genitourinary clinic, *Critical Public Health.* **10**(3): 1–17.

Pryce A (2005) ... planting landmines in their sex lives: Governmentality, iconography of sexual disease and the 'duties' of the STD clinic. In King M and Watson K (eds) *Representing Health: Discourses of Health and illness in the Media.* Palgrave, London, pp. 156–183.

Raftery J (1996) The decline of the asylum or the poverty of the concept?. In Tomlinson D and Carrier J (eds.) *Asylum in the Community.* Routledge, London, pp. 18–30.

Rankin J (2001) Texts in action: How nurses are doing the fiscal work of health care reform. *Studies in Cultures, Organizations, and Societies.* **7**(2): 251–267.

Rayner S (1986) Management of radiation hazards in hospitals: plural rationalities in a single institution. *Social Studies of Science.* **16**(4): 573–591.

Read J (2000) *Disability, the Family and Society.* Open University Press, Buckingham.

Redfern S and Ross F M (1999) Reflections. In Redfern S and Ross F (eds) *Nursing Older People* (3rd edn). Churchill Livingstone, London, pp. 619–631.

Reed J (1998) Care and protection for older people. In Heyman, B (ed.) *Risk, Health and Health Care: A Qualitative Approach.* Edward Arnold, London, pp. 241–251.

Ridge D (2004) 'It was an incredible thrill': The social meanings and dynamics of younger gay men's experiences of barebacking in Melbourne. *Sexualities.* **7**(3): 259–279.

Rietmeijer C A, Bull S S and McFarlane M (2001) Sex and the Internet. *AIDS.* **15**(11):1433–1434.

Ritchie Inquiry (1994) *Report of the Inquiry into the Care and Treatment of Christopher Clunis,* Chairman J H Ritchie. HMSO, London.

Roberts G and Holly J (1996) *Risk Management in Healthcare.* Witherby, London.

Roberts S J (1983) Oppressed group behaviour: implications for nursing. *Advances in Nursing Science.* 5(July): 21–30.

Rolfe G (1998) *Expanding Nursing Knowledge: Understanding and Researching Your Own Practice.* Butterworth Heinemann, Oxford.

Rose N (1990) *Governing the Soul: The Shaping of the Private Self.* Routledge, London.

—— (1993) Government, authority and expertise in advanced liberalism. *Economy and Society.* **22**(3): 283–299.

Rose N (1996) Psychiatry as a political science: advanced liberalism and the administration of risk. *History of Human Sciences.* **9**(2): 1–23.

—— (1998) Governing risky individuals: the role of psychiatry in new regimes of control. *Psychiatry, Psychology and Law.* **5**(2): 177–195.

—— (1998) Living dangerously: risk-thinking and risk management in mental health care. *Mental Health Care.* **1**(8): 263–266.

—— (2000) Government and control. *British Journal of Criminology.* **40**(2): 321–339.

Rosengren W R and DeVault S (1963) The sociology of time and space in an obstetric hospital. In Freidson E (ed.) *The Hospital in Modern Society.* The Free Press, New York, pp. 266–292.

Rosenstock I (1974) Historical origins of the health belief model. In Becker M (ed.) *The Health Belief Model and Personal Behavior.* Charles B. Slack, Thorofare, NJ, pp. 1–8.

Roth J A (1957) Ritual and magic in the Control of Contagion. *American Sociological Review.* **22**(3): 310–314.

Rothman D J (1971) *The Discovery of the Asylum.* Mass, Little, Brown and Co., Boston.

Royal College of Nursing (RCN)(1998) *Dealing with Violence Towards Nursing Staff.* RCN, London.

—— (2002) *Working Well? Results from the RCN Working Well Survey into the Wellbeing and Working Lives of Nurses.* (RCN), London, 001 572.

Royal College of Nursing Institute (2004) *The Picture of a Life-Study Guide.* Royal College of Nursing Institute, London.

Royal College of Paediatrics & Child Health (2002) *Immunisation of the Immuno-compromised Child: Best Practice Statement.* Royal College of Paediatrics & Child Health, London.

Ryan J W and Spellbring A M (1996) Implementing strategies to decrease risk of falls in older women. *Journal of Gerontological Nursing.* **22**(12): 25–31.

Saunders M (1998) Management of risk. In Pickering S and Thompson J S (eds) *Promoting Positive Practice in Nursing Older People.* Bailliere Tindall, London, pp. 72–89.

Saurel-Cubizolles M J, Zeitlin J, Lelong N, Papiernik E, Di Renzo G C and Breart G (2004) Employment, working conditions, and preterm birth: results for the Europop case-control survey. *J Epidemiol Community Health.* **58**(39): 395–401.

Schön D A (1988) From Technical Rationality to Reflection-in-Action. In Dowie J and Elstein A (eds) *Professional Judgment, A Reader in Clinical Decision Making,* Cambridge University Press, Cambridge.

Scott J (2000) *Understanding Contemporary Society: Theories of The Present,* Browning G, Halcli A and Webster F (eds) Sage, London.

Sharkey P (2000) *The Essentials of Community Care*. Macmillan, London.

Shaw F, Bond J and Richardson (2003) Multi-factoral intervention after a fall in older people with cognitive impairment and dementia presenting to the accident and emergency department: Randomised controlled trial. *British Medical Journal*. **326**(7380): 73–85.

Shirtliffe D (1995) Risk-taking for clients with learning disabilities. *Nursing Times*. **91**(5): 40–42.

Shore C, Austin J and Dunn D (2004) Maternal adaptation to a child's epilepsy. *Epilepsy & Behaviour*. **5**(4): 557–568.

Simon W (1996) *Postmodern Sexualities*. Routledge, London.

Simon W and Gagnon J H (1999) Sexual scripts. In Parker R and Aggleton P (eds) *Culture, Society & Sexuality*. University College London Press, London, pp. 29–38.

Simpson M (1994) Here come the mirror men, *The Independent*, November 15, (www.wordspy.com/words/metrosexual.asp Accessed: June 2005)

Sines D (1995) Impaired autonomy – the challenge of caring ... changing power relationships between learning disability nurses and their clients. *Journal of Clinical Nursing*. **4**(2): 109–115.

Skolbekken J A (1995) The risk epidemic in medical journals. *Social Science & Medicine*. **40**(3): 291–305.

Smith D E (1987) *The Everyday World as Problematic: A Feminist Sociology*. University of Toronto Press, Toronto.

—— (1990) *The Conceptual Practices of Power: A Feminist Sociology of Knowledge*. Routledge, New York.

—— (1999) *Writing the Social: Critique, Theory, Investigations*. University of Toronto Press, Toronto.

—— (2001) Texts and the ontology of organizations and institutions. *Studies in Cultures, Organizations and Societies*. **7**(2): 147–198.

—— (2002) Institutional ethnography. In Tim May (ed.) *Qualitative research in action.*: Sage, Thousand Oaks, CA, pp. 17–52.

Society of Obstetricians and Gynaecologists of Canada. (2000). *Healthy Beginnings: Your Handbook for Pregnancy and Birth* (2nd edn). SOGC, Ottawa.

Sontag S (1988) *AIDS and its Metaphors*. Penguin, London.

Stanko E A (1996) Reading danger: sexual harassment, anticipation and self-protection. In Hester M, Kelly L and Radford J (eds) *Women, Violence and Male Power*. Open University Press, Buckingham, pp. 50–62.

Stevens-Simon C and Orleans M (1999) Low-birthweight prevention programs: The enigma of failure. *Birth*. **26**(3): 184–191.

Stewart P J (1998) Primary prevention of preterm birth. *Preterm Birth Prevention Conference.* 24th to 25th April 1998, Ottawa.

Storr M (1999) Postmodern bisexuality. *Sexualities.* 2(3): 309–325.

Strombeck R (2003) Finding sex partners on-line: A new high-risk practice among older adults? *JAIDS Journal of Acquired Immune Deficiency Syndromes.* 33(Supplement 2): 226–228.

Suter G (1993) *Ecological risk assessment.* Lewis, Chelsea, Oklahoma.

Swift P and Pontin D (2001) Care Management and Community Nursing. In Hyde V (ed.) *Community Nursing and Health Care: Insights and Innovations.* Arnold, London, pp. 119–137.

Swartz D (1997) *Culture and Power: The Sociology of Pierre Bourdieu.* University of Chicago Press, Chicago.

Tew M (1990) *Safer Childbirth: A Critical History of Maternity Care.* Chapman Hall, London.

Tinetti M E and Powell L (1993) Fear of falling and low self-efficacy: A cause of dependence in elderly persons. *Journal of Gerontology.* 48(Special Issue): 35–38.

The Internet's Resource for Addiction (www.radat.bc.ca/index.php? C=internet-addiction&T=addiction-internet-sex Accessed: June 2005)

Tomaney J (1994) A new paradigm of work organization and technology. In Amin A (ed.) *Post-Fordism: A Reader.* Blackwell, Oxford, pp. 157–194.

Townsend E (1998) *Good Intentions Overruled: A Critique of Empowerment in the Routine Organization of Mental Health Services.* University of Toronto Press, Toronto.

Trenoweth S (2003) Perceiving risk in dangerous situations: risks of violence among mental health patients. *Journal of Advanced Nursing.* 42(3): 278–287.

Tuke S (1964) *Desrciption of the Retreat: An Instituition Near York, for Insane Persons of the Society of Friends,* with and introduction by Hunter R and MacAlpine I. Dawsons, London.

Tulloch J and Lupton D (2003) *Risk and Everyday Life.* Sage, London.

United Kingdom Central Council for Nursing, Midwifery and Health Visiting (UKCC) (2002) *The Recognition, Prevention and Therapeutic Management of Violence in Mental Health Care: A Summary. A Initiative Supported by the Government Health Departments and the Statutory Mental Health Bodies in the Four Countries of the United Kingdom.* UKCC, London.

Upson A (2004) *Violence at Work: Findings from the 2002/2003 British Crime Survey: Home Office Online Report 04/04.* Home Office, London.

Van Dongen-Melman J, Van Zuuren F and Verhulst F (1998) Experiences of parents of childhood cancer survivors: a qualitative analysis. *Patient Education & Counselling* 34(3): 185–200.

Van Kemenade S (2003) Social Capital as a Health Determinant: How is it Defined? (www.hc-sc.ca/arad-draa. Accessed: June 2004)

Vissandjee B, Desmeules M, Cao Z and Abdool S (2004) Integrating socio-economic determinants of Canadian women's health. *BMC Women's Health* 4(Supplement 1), S34. (www. biomedcentral.com/1472-6874/4/S1/S34. Accessed: September 2004)

Vos M (2005) Speech summary (www.dh.gov.uk/NewsHome/ ConferenceAndEventReports/ConferenceReportsConference ReportsArticle/fs/en?CONTENT_ID=4102049&chk=GgHAE H. Accessed: February 2005)

Wacquant L (1995) Pugs at work: bodily capital and bodily labour among professional boxers. *Body & Society* 1(1): 65–93.

Walters V (2004) The social context of women's health. BMC Women's Health, 4(Suppl 1), S2. (www.biomedcentral.com/ 1472-6874/4/S1/S2. Accessed: September 2004)

Weber M (1948) Bureaucracy. In Gerth H H and Wright Mills C (eds) *From Max Weber: Essays in Sociology.* Routledge & Kegan Paul, London. pp. 196–244.

Weeks J (2000) *Making Sexual History.* Polity Press, Cambridge.

Weiss M E, Saks N P and Harris S (2002) Resolving the uncertainty of preterm symptoms: Women's experiences with the onset of preterm labor. *Journal of Obstetric, Gynecologic, and Neonatal Nursing.* 31(1): 66–76.

Wells G (1996) *Hazard Iidentification and Risk Assessment.* Institute of Chemical Engineers, Rugby.

Wells J and Bowers L (2002) How prevalent is violence towards nurses working in general hospitals in the UK? *Journal of Advanced Nursing.* 39(3): 230–240.

Welsh S, Hassiotis A, O'Mahoney G and Deahl M (2003) Big brother is watching you: The ethical implications of electronic surveillance measures in the elderly with dementia and in adults with learning difficulties. *Aging & Mental Health.* 7(5): 372–375.

Wergeland E and Strand K (1998) Need for job adjustment in pregnancy: Early prediction based on work history. *Scandinavian Journal of Primary Health Care.* 16(2): 90–94.

White K (2002) *An Introduction to the Sociology of Health and Illness.* Sage, London.

Whitfield L (2003) Catch them if he can: the interview- Jim Gee. *Health Service Journal.* **113** (5877)(16 October): 30–31.

Whittaker A and McIntosh B (2000) Changing days. *British Journal of Learning Disabilities.* **28**(1): 3–8.

Whittington R, Shuttleworth S and Hill L (1996) Violence to staff in a general hospital setting. *Journal of Advanced Nursing.* **24**(2): 326–333.

Willams J, Steel C, Sharp G, DelosReyes E, Phillips T, Bates S, Lange B and Griebel M (2003) Parental anxiety and quality of life in children with epilepsy. *Epilepsy & Behaviour* **4**(5): 483–486.

Winstanley S and Whittington R (2002) Violence in a general hospital: comparison of assailant and other assault-related factors on accident and emergency and inpatient wards. *Acta Psychiatrica Scandinavica.*106 (Supplement): 144–147.

Winstanley S and Whittington R (2004) Aggression towards health care staff in a UK general hospital: Variation Among Professions and Departments. *Journal of Clinical Nursing.* **13**(1): 3–10.

Wolfensberger W. (1972) *The Principle of Normalisation in Human Services.* Leonard Crainford, Toronto.

World Health Organization (1975) *Education and Treatment in Human Sexuality: The Training Of Health Professionals* (www2.hu-berlin.de/sexology/GESUND/ARCHIV/ WHOR.HTM#N3 Accessed: June 2005)

World Health Organization (2002) *Working Definition of Sexual Health* (www.who.int/reproductive-health/gender/sexual_ health.html Accessed: June 2005)

Wright S, Gray R, Parkes J and Gournay K (2002) *The Recognition, Prevention and Therapeutic Management of Violence in Acute In-Patient Psychiatry: A Literature Review and Evidence-Based Recommendations for Good Practice. Prepared for the United Kingdom Central Council for Nursing, Midwifery and Health Visiting.* UKCC & Institute of Psychiatry, London.

Wynne B (1992) Risk and social learning: reification to engagement. In Krimsky S & Golding D (eds) *Social Theories of Risk.* Praeger, Westport, Colorado, pp. 275–300.

Wynne R, Clarkin N, Cox T and Griffiths A (1997) *Guidance on the Prevention of Violence at Work.* European Commission, Luxembourg.

Wynne-Harley D (1991) *Living Dangerously: Risk-taking, Safety and Older People.* Centre for Policy on Ageing, London.

Name index

Subject index